FASTING
CAN CHANGE
YOUR LIFE

⋛ JERRY FALWELL AND ELMER TOWNS ⋚
EDITORS

THE STORIES OF MANY WHO FAST,
including:
JERRY FALWELL
BILL BRIGHT
JACK HAYFORD
CINDY JACOBS
D. JAMES KENNEDY
JIMMY DRAPER
JANE HANSEN
BILL GREIG JR.
EVELYN CHRISTENSON
RONNIE FLOYD
ELMER TOWNS

Regal

A Division of Gospel Light
Ventura, California, U.S.A.

Published by Regal Books
A Division of Gospel Light
Ventura, California, U.S.A.
Printed in U.S.A.

Regal Books is a ministry of Gospel Light, an evangelical Christian publisher dedicated to serving the local church. We believe God's vision for Gospel Light is to provide church leaders with biblical, user-friendly materials that will help them evangelize, disciple and minister to children, youth and families.

It is our prayer that this Regal book will help you discover biblical truth for your own life and help you meet the needs of others. May God richly bless you.

For a free catalog of resources from Regal Books and Gospel Light please call your Christian supplier, or contact us at 1-800-4-GOSPEL or at www.gospellight.com.

Cover Design by Kevin Keller
Interior Design by Britt Rocchio
Edited by Virginia Woodard

Library of Congress Cataloging-in-Publication Data
Fasting can change your life / Jerry Falwell and Elmer Towns,
   editors.
      p. cm.
   Includes index.
   ISBN 0-8307-2197-5 (pbk.)
   1. Fasting. I. Falwell, Jerry. II. Towns, Elmer L.
   BV5055.W47 1998   98-34361
   248.4 7—dc21   CIP

1 2 3 4 5 6 7 8 9 10 11 12 13 14 15 16 17 18 19 20 / 04 03 02 01 00 99 98

Rights for publishing this book in other languages are contracted by
Gospel Literature International (GLINT). GLINT also provides technical help for the adaptation, translation and publishing of Bible study resources and books in scores of languages worldwide. For further information, contact GLINT, P.O. Box 4060, Ontario, CA 91761-1003, U.S.A., or the publisher. You may also send e-mail to Glintint@aol.com, or visit their web site at www.glint.org.

⋗ WARNING: ⋖

The fasts suggested in this book are not for everyone. Consult your physician before beginning. Expectant mothers, diabetics and others who have a history of medical problems can enter the spirit of fasting while remaining on essential diets. Although fasting is healthful to many, the nature of God would not command a physical exercise that would harm people physically or emotionally.

Liberty University has established a Founder's Chair for the School of Religion. We are pleased that funds to begin the endowment have been pledged from a number of sources, including Jerry Falwell and Elmer Towns. They have assigned the copyright, royalties and other compensation coming from their book to endow the Founder's Chair.

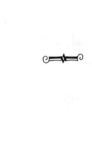

⇉ CONTENTS ⇇

Some fast privately, as Jane Hansen did, agonizing for a son addicted to drugs. God heard, the son was saved and was delivered from addiction to drugs. Some fast corporately and publicly: 5,000 students at Liberty University shut down the food service center because they dedicated a day to pray for Dean of Students Vernon Brewer's healing from cancer. The congregation of St. Peter's Lutheran Church in Fort Pierce, Florida, was able to sell their property after fasting for a sale.

Jimmy Draper, president of The Sunday School Board of the Southern Baptist Convention, was so touched by God that he could not eat for days. To him, fasting was not to receive something, but he fasted for a week *after* experiencing the presence of Christ and God's assurance of salvation. Gene Mims, a vice president, did not want to accept a position at the Sunday School Board of the Southern Baptist Convention until he fasted, and in that experience knew God was calling him to a new area of service. Larry Boan, a staff pastor at an Assembly of God church, committed himself to fast 40 days for the salvation of his dying father. He was able to witness his father's conversion a few days before his death.

The Hebrew term fasting (*tsom*) originally was associated with emergency or distress; people were losing their appetites because of anguish or fear. When we rush to the hospital because a loved one had an accident, we do not consider pulling into McDonald's for a hamburger because it is lunchtime. The emergency pushes the thought of food out of our minds. All we want to do is fix the problem. When a problem is bigger than life, many may fast until it is solved.

Gary Greig, who earned a Ph.D. in Hebrew from one of the most prestigious institutions in the world, Chicago University, rid himself of fear by fasting.

Fasting was originally commanded of God's people on the Day of Atonement, a fasting day for the Jews. Now, a one-day fast is called by its Hebrew term, a Yom Kippur Fast. Many fasted from sundown to sundown, following God's designation He gave in Genesis 1:5: "The evening and the morning were the first day." During mealtime of that day they fasted and prayed instead of eating. Fasting does not become effective when we stop eating; it begins when we start praying. Our effectiveness in fasting is measured by our ability to touch God and be touched by Him.

Study carefully what people drink when they fast. (It is important not to go without liquids for more than one to three days, as brain damage can occur from dehydration and/or loss of liquids.) Some drink only water, as did Jerry Falwell; some blend fruit and/or vegetables into a drink. Some drink Slim-Fast, others Ensure, both commercial products. Falwell says fruit or vegetable drinks are not acceptable; he only drinks nonnutrients. On the other hand, some won't drink fruit juice, because they like it, saying the rule should be that what they drink should be unenjoyable.

After interviewing many who have fasted successfully, however, it seems God looks at the heart, not the liquid intake. He answers many prayers, recognizing many expressions of fasting. Remember the law of silence: *When God has not spoken, don't make rules.* So we should not make rules about what others should or should not drink during a fast. Before we criticize them, we should try going 40 days or 7 days just drinking Slim Fast or Ensure or juice. We should let the Holy Spirit lead us in what to drink. First, it is important to immerse ourselves in Scripture; second, yield our understanding to God; third, follow the urgings from the Holy Spirit.

Fasting is hard, especially for the first two or three days. After that it becomes physically easier, but the mental pressure begins to build. After a while our bodies do not demand food, but the pressure from our families can be strong. They are eating, why can't we? We may have to attend luncheon meetings, banquets and prayer breakfasts where everyone but us is eating. This is tough during a fast.

In the presence of God, however, we do not think about physical food; we feast spiritually on God. When we are talking to God, we forget about eating anything.

We may fast when prayer is not enough to receive the answers we need. We may fast for an emergency, something that could destroy us, and we are scared. Jerry Falwell thought he might lose the University he began, so he fasted for 40 days; but God told him not to ask for money. God impressed on Falwell to get his focus right and to position himself for an answer. Falwell ended the 40-day fast without his answer, and began eating again. Twenty-five days later, God impressed upon him to fast and pray for money. He entered another 40-day fast (he did not eat for 80 days out of 105 days and lost 82 pounds), then God gave the University $27 million dollars and other things necessary to stave off bankruptcy and loss of accreditation. Liberty University had all sanctions removed by the accreditation agency and was voted reaffirmation for another 10 years.

Others fasted for healing, such as Cindy Jacobs, Les Ayars and David Rhodenhizer.

Troy Temple fasted when he and his wife could not produce children. Did God answer their request by granting fertilization? No! However, during the time Troy was fasting, in another place, a young lady conceived, and the Temples were able to adopt this child a little more than nine months later.

This book was not intended to be a practical manual about fasting, but you will learn many *how-to* principles to make your fast more meaningful. Watch for the "Take-Aways" section at the end of each testimony. They are a summary of a great lesson you can learn from that particular testimony.

Many of these stories are included to stretch your faith and to challenge you by their examples. If you are discouraged about the work of God in your life or church, this book is written to challenge you to fast about it. If you will trust God for greater things, then this book has served its purpose.

Notice the kind of stories we have included. We have included a few stories about fasting for money or church buildings to challenge you to fast for things. We have included a few great illustrations of healing through fasting to inspire you. We have included a few reports of fasting for the salvation of lost people to challenge you to fast and pray for those who are lost.

Notice also that we have included testimonies of well-known Christian leaders such as Bill Bright and D. James Kennedy, though fasting is not just for those who are in the spotlight. We have included the stories of lesser-known believers who took a step of faith—even when it was not in the spotlight. Lesser-known believers, however, took steps unknown to others—and God answered.

The stories were read by each interviewee to ensure reliability. We did not include all the stories of those we interviewed, but chose those that best reflected the areas where believers fast and pray. Thank you to each for allowing us to include a glimpse of your life in this book.

All royalties for this book go to Liberty University to train young champions for Christ and not to the editors or individuals whose stories are told.

May the testimonies of this book challenge us all to know Christ and make Him known.

Sincerely yours in Christ,
Jerry Falwell and Elmer Towns
The Editors

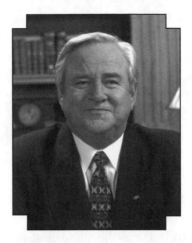

JERRY FALWELL

Pastor, Thomas Road Baptist Church, Lynchburg, Virginia
Chancellor, Liberty University
Founder, Moral Majority Inc., Lynchburg, Virginia

Of all the organizations Jerry Falwell has founded, he wants to be introduced as pastor of Thomas Road Baptist Church, a 22,000-member church he began in 1956 and has pastored for 42 years. Although some have gone on to other pursuits, Jerry, as most of his members call him, still makes hospital calls, performs weddings and funerals, and preaches most of the sermons.

The vast influence of Jerry Falwell springs from his church, which gave birth to the "Old Time Gospel Hour." He also founded Liberty University, which has 14,000 students in attendance, Liberty Baptist Theological Seminary, Liberty Bible Institute, Elim Home for alcoholic men, the Godparent Home for pregnant single girls, and Moral Majority, the platform from which he gathers political reputation.

The awards are many for Falwell, from honorary doctorate degrees to the *Good Housekeeping* magazine's "10 Most Admired Men in America" to being featured on the covers of *Time* and *Newsweek* magazines. He has counseled privately Presidents Nixon, Reagan and Bush, as well as other world leaders.

Perhaps his greatest influence is that more than 2,000 graduates of Liberty University pastor churches, of which approximately 600 have planted churches. More than 800 graduates serve as foreign missionaries.

The greatness of Falwell is seen in his love for Christ as evidenced in two 40-day fasts within 105 days, which brought more than $52 million and renewed accreditation to Liberty University.

1

GETTING 50 MILLION DOLLARS

Interview with

JERRY FALWELL

FAVORITE VERSE ABOUT FASTING:

I am the Lord thy God, which brought thee out of the land of Egypt: open thy mouth wide, and I will fill it.
—*Psalm 81:10*

Question: Tell me the first time you ever fasted.

Falwell: I was converted at age 18. In those days there was not much preaching on fasting and prayer, but I heard enough to know that in a time of crisis, fasting with prayer could be helpful to get answers from God. So with my limited understanding as a new convert, I did go on a few one-day fasts. I would always fast after dinner the first day until dinner the following day. I would abstain from breakfast and lunch, a practice I learned then and have done from time to time to the present day. Usually these one-day fasts are based on personal challenges or needs in the lives of people who are close to me.

Question: You began calling your church to fast about the time you began Liberty University. Describe those events.

Falwell: In the early days of Liberty, it was a common thing for our church to fast for the University. We were building three or four buildings a year during the late '70s and early '80s. We were paying cash as we built. We never borrowed long-term money until many years after that. Yet it was not uncommon for me to ask the University and church families to fast and pray for an entire day for the provision of large sums of money: a million dollars, five million dollars, whatever was needed for construction at that time. We always fasted from solid food, except for nonnutrient liquids. We would begin after an evening meal of literally eating nothing with nutrient value until dinner the next day.

Question: You usually called a fast on Monday, beginning sundown after the evening church services. Why did you do that?

Falwell: I would usually ask the people to fast after church on Sunday until before dinner on Monday because I had the entire Lord's Day, morning and night, to challenge and encourage the people to unite in a corporate fast. Human beings are very busy today and are entangled with personal and business affairs. When I have challenged them to fast on days other than Monday, they have good intentions to fast, but because there is no one on Wednesday or Thursday night saying, "OK, let's do it," the percentage of involvement is not very high.

Question: Did you fast for the healing of Charles Hughes?

Falwell: Yes, the whole University and church family fasted for Charles's healing in 1978. I was in Holland, Michigan, preaching when the accident happened. Charles was unconscious for 14 days. His father, Dr. Robert Hughes, came and asked me to call a day of fasting and prayer throughout the entire ministry. We did do that.

Charles was an upperclassman at Liberty University with great potential. God had called Charles to preach and serve Him. Charles was so gifted that we used him in the "I Love America" crusades. This was a crusade where I preached on the capitol steps of almost every state capitol building in America. As a student, in each crusade Charles gave a patriotic reading that was powerfully used by God.

On the way to an evangelistic crusade in Harrisburg, Pennsylvania, where he was scheduled to preach, the van in which he was riding was mangled in an accident with an 18-wheel truck. Charles's head was crushed, and they removed the top of his skull because of swelling. The doctors told us Charles would die and asked if the family would sign papers to donate some of his body organs to living recipients. The medical community felt Charles was as good as dead.

Question: Describe the statement of faith you made.

Falwell: I told everyone Charles would live if we deeply fasted and prayed from the depths of our hearts. I was so sure that God would answer our prayers that I announced Charles was going to speak at Liberty's graduation that year.

Charles lived and was restored enough to bring a powerful message at the 1978 graduation. Liberty had previously had well-known speakers such as Dr. W. A. Criswell of First Baptist Church, Dallas, Texas, and Dr. Charles Stanley, pastor of First Baptist Church, Atlanta, Georgia, but to me the greatness of that message was not what Charles said, but the testimony of his healing as he stood before the audience that day.

Question: Describe the fast for Vernon Brewer on April 25, 1985.

Falwell: I was at the hospital when the doctor approached Patty Brewer and the family to advise them that the tumor was very large and his condition was very grave. I don't recall the specific events prior to that fast, but probably those two events, fasting for Charles Hughes and Vernon Brewer, commanded more prayer attention and fasting than any other individuals in my 41 years in the ministry. And in both cases, they survived.

Vernon Brewer was dean of students and vice president at Liberty University in 1985. Vernon was a graduate of Liberty in our first graduating class. The students loved Vernon because of his fairness in enforcing rules and his deep love for them. I knew that more than 5,000 students joined me to pray and fast for Vernon. God healed him. That demonstrated to me the power of corporate fasting and prayer. Today, Vernon leads the World Help organization. God is using him to reach the world through a foreign-missions outreach organization. (See chapter 11 for complete details.)

Question: Describe your 40-day fast. What were the events that led up to this fast?

Falwell: Liberty University had no long-term debt on its property in 1986. I raised the money on television for whatever buildings or projects were needed. Also, we raised funds by direct mail. We never had difficulty raising cash to build Liberty University. Liberty was the fastest-growing Christian school in the world. We had raised more than $27 million of needed cash every year. But when Jim Bakker and Jim Swaggart fell and drew such media attention, it became clear by the late '80s that we could no longer raise money through television appeals, or support the University financially by direct mail. Because of the national religious scandals, the evangelical religious community would never be the same again.

I often compare television ministries to what happened in the savings and loan industry. When the bad ones began falling like dominoes, many good savings and loans were wiped out in the tidal wave. Likewise, many strong evangelical media ministries such as ours were permanently hurt. People stopped giving because of a credibility crunch. Giving went down substantially in our ministry and other ministries. Contributions to the "Old Time Gospel Hour" and Liberty University went down about $25 million a year, which was about 25 percent of our total revenue.

We had a university, we had buildings constructed, we had

spent about $250 million on facilities, but suddenly we found ourselves unable to raise money to pay bills. After four consecutive years of $25 million deficits, we suddenly had $100 million to $110 million in liability debt. We had students on campus and we couldn't send them home.

The first thing I did was to dismantle the Moral Majority, got out of the political ring and came back to Lynchburg in November 1991 to concentrate all my energies on Liberty University. I moved my office for the first time onto the campus of Liberty. It was through days and nights of fasting and prayer. . . just to raise enough to pay our electric bill or meet salaries. It was a monumental task of restoring the school to financial stability. From 1991 to 1996, I practiced fasting and prayer as never before in my personal life. Survival was the name of the game. Finally, at the end of the fiscal year, June 30, 1996, by God's enablement, the debt had been reduced from $110 million by more than $70 million.

Besides the financial debt, a double-barreled shotgun was pointed at our head with both hammers cocked. Liberty University was threatened with losing its regional accreditation. Because the Southern Association of Colleges and Schools would not reaffirm accreditation for a university that had such precarious indebtedness as ours, Liberty had to reduce its debt before it could continue its accredited status. SACS (Southern Association of Colleges and Schools) put Liberty on probation in December 1996. Without accreditation, I didn't think the University could continue. With this crisis, I had to fast, and fast seriously.

And the Lord impressed upon my heart in the summer of 1996 that it was time to do the unthinkable, that is, personally go on an absolute 40-day fast. From July 20 to the first of September, I fasted and prayed that 1997-1998 would be the year when Liberty's debt burden was removed by God. So I fasted 40 days, July 20 through September 1. I saw mighty things beginning to happen, but I wasn't really sure. In that first fast of 40 days, I kept asking

God for money, but He impressed upon my heart that I needed to get close to Him, to listen to Him and to trust Him. When I asked for money, God told me not to ask for money, but to learn to know Him better. I had several lessons to learn before I could ask for money. As I ended that first 40-day fast, I felt I had learned what God wanted to teach me. But I didn't have an answer about money.

After resuming my normal diet for 25 days, God told me I could ask Him for money. So I went back on another 40-day fast that began September 25, 1996, ending on November 4. I broke the fast that evening. I had fasted for 80 days out of 105 days during the summer and fall.

I was in Nashville, Tennessee, preaching at Two Rivers Baptist Church at a God Save America rally. We went out for a light meal; it was my first meal in 40 days.

Question: What were the tangible results of that fast?

Falwell: First, we received a cash gift large enough to pay off our long-term mortgage debt. Second, we replenished the cash flow of Liberty University with several million dollars that gave us financial and institutional health. Third, God sent Liberty a new president, Dr. John Borek, a Ph.D. in business administration, who had been the chief financial officer at Georgia State University. Without him we might not have been prepared for SACS's accreditation visit. Fourth, when SACS visited and then evaluated Liberty, they removed all sanctions and recommended Liberty University for 10 years of reaffirmation, which is the bottom line of why I fasted.

One individual has given Liberty University close to $50 million since those two fasts. And so those two 40-day fasts were unlike any experiences I have ever had.

Question: What did you eat or drink during your two 40-day fasts?

Falwell: On July 15, 1996, I went to Dr. Gregg Albers, my doctor, and told him I was thinking about a 40-day fast. He said I had to have fluids. I told him I was going to use water only, but he said, "I would recommend that every few days you take a small glass of fruit or vegetable juice," so I chose V-8. About every third or fourth day I would drink an 8-ounce glass of V-8. Every day I drank a lot of water . . . a lot of water. To me it is not a fast if you're drinking blended food or drinking any kind of food value. I also took one Centrum, a vitamin tablet, every morning. After about 10 days, the hunger pangs subsided and about the thirty-fifth day they returned. The last five days were the hardest struggle. In the middle of the fast there was a spiritual release. During those two fasts, I lost 82 pounds.

Question: What about loss of energy?

Falwell: I noticed no substantial loss of energy. The last five days of both fasts I found myself becoming weary in the evening.

TAKE-AWAYS

The greater the problem, the greater dedication you have to make to get an answer from God. The longer lasting a problem, the longer you have to fast and pray for an answer. When the problem becomes life threatening to you or to your ministry, you must make a greater sacrifice of physical pleasure or even physical well-being until you get an answer from God.

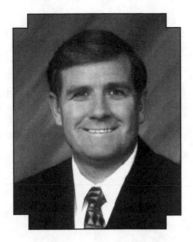

AL HENSON

Pastor, Lighthouse Baptist Church
Greater Nashville, Tennessee

One of the largest and fastest-growing churches planted by a Liberty graduate is also considered by many the strongest spiritually. Al Henson left Liberty Baptist Theological Seminary in 1978 and immediately began Lighthouse Baptist Church in the recreation room of an apartment complex. Because he believes God intervenes in the problems that face the work of God, he fasted and prayed for 25 acres of ground on Interstate 24. The provision of the ground was miraculous.

When Henson went to Nashville, he did not pray for hundreds. "I prayed for one family a week." During that first year, 53 families joined the church. As a matter of fact, everyone prayed for a family a week to join the church. Sometimes when a family visited the church, someone said to them, "You're the family we have been praying for."

Lighthouse Baptist Church and Christian School received an annual income of $3.5 million in 1997, and the school has 725 students. They have constructed five buildings for a total worth of $5 million in assets. Henson also began the Lighthouse Baptist College. The church averages almost 800 in weekly attendance, has helped plant 15 new churches in five states and now has more than 25 Liberty graduates working for the church or as evangelists and/or church planters. Liberty University honored Al Henson with the doctor of divinity degree.

2

RECEIVING
24 ACRES FOR
A NEW CHURCH

Interview with
AL HENSON

FAVORITE VERSE ABOUT FASTING:

And Jesus said unto them, Can the children of the
bridechamber mourn, as long as the bridegroom is with
them? but the days will come, when the bridegroom shall
be taken from them, and then shall they fast.
—*Matthew 9:15*

Question: How did God first lead you into the ministry of fasting?

Henson: When I first came to seminary at Liberty, it was my heart passion to know the Lord. My life verse is Philippians 3:10, "That I may know him, and the power of his resurrection." And as I began to study the Bible, I felt fasting was one of the most effective ways to set time aside to seek God, that I might find God and that I may know Him.

Question: What was your practice of fasting at seminary?

Henson: Since the very beginning of my seminary days, I've had a goal to fast at least one day every week. I've continued that discipline even to this point. A lot of people look at fasting as a means of getting things. I've never fasted to receive an answer to prayer; I made the primary purpose of my fasting to seek God that I might know Him. My wife and I went to the prayer chapel at Thomas Road Baptist Church on the afternoon of the day we fasted (usually Wednesdays) for two hours of prayer. We not only wanted to know Christ, but we were also fasting and praying for the church we planned to start in Nashville, Tennessee.

Question: How did your faith grow?

Henson: When I was a student at Liberty, I wanted to put God to the test. I wanted to see a miracle so I would know that God's provision would be available in starting a new church. I had $1,057. I paid a $17 water bill, $40 for groceries and gave $1,000 to the church. I did not tell my wife or anyone else. I asked God to provide for our needs. God moved a couple to Thomas Road Baptist Church, close friends I now call "Mom and Pop Morris," who felt led to help a student through school. They invited us to move into their home, giving us a place to live without rent, plus helping us purchase food. I figure that the Morrises gave us more than $7,000 worth of rent and groceries, seven times the amount I had given to God.

Question: How did fasting help plant a new church?

Henson: When the church was only two months old, I passed 25 acres on Interstate 24 not far from the apartment building where I was living. As I drove past and saw the tenement house, I knew the property might be purchased. When I first contacted the owner, he refused to sell the land because he planned to will the property to his daughter. When I called on the owner a second time, I was told, "No!" emphatically. I walked the property line and prayed for the tract of land. On several occasions I returned and knelt on the property and asked God to give it to us. I believed that God would give the land to the church.

Finally, for three days, I fasted and prayed that God would touch the owner's heart. I got the church to pray for the property with me. Then I visited the man and shared my burden for reaching the city of Nashville. As I left, I asked the owner, "Will you pray about selling the property to us?" Before he could answer, the man's wife said, "I'll see that he prays about it."

The next morning while I was shaving, the man phoned me and said, "The Lord spoke to me as I have never had Him speak to me before; I know that God wants you to have this property." Then he went on, "If you will come up with $29,000, I will loan you the other $71,000 to buy the property." (The property was valued at $175,000. The owner eliminated the first $75,000 off the value as a gift.) The church was given 90 days to raise the down payment on the mortgage that was pegged at 9 percent interest.

Slowly some money came in. Six days before the deadline, the church had raised only $5,000. A Christian friend, Malcolm Barrett, not a member of the church, told me, "I have been listening to you on the radio." He invited me, "Let's get on our knees and pray about this money." After praying, he said, "Come by tomorrow and I will get $24,000 for the property." He loaned the church the money at no interest for an indefinite period. This was one of the greatest miracles in the life of the church.

I would not want to leave the impression that I fasted to get that property. I was fasting to know the will of the Lord, and once I knew the will of God, I knew He would carry out His will.

Question: When your church was getting ready to build your present church, didn't you go on a fast in a small tent up on the hill where the auditorium was built? Tell the story.

Henson: I felt the number-one need was to have the assurance that God wanted us to move ahead with the construction. Second, that if we did move ahead with the construction, I wanted the assurance that the Lord would bless and empower the ministry on that piece of property. So I picked a place as close as I could to where the building would be located when finished. I pitched the tent and lived there for 21 days. I would come down an hour a day to the church office to handle necessary business. Basically, my staff took care of everything, but at a set hour each day, I would come down and meet with the pastors.

My wife and children would come and visit with me on a day-to-day basis. I had some hours each day when anyone from the church could come up and pray with me. Apart from those hours, I was alone. I stayed there for 21 days; actually, it extended into 22 days because after 21 days I still didn't have a definite peace from God. On the twenty-second day of fasting, praying and seeking the Lord, I was getting weak.

I remember walking down through the trees, stumbling and falling. I fell flat, my face landed in the dirt. I remembered at that moment God surrounded me and said, "You are released." God seemed to impress upon my soul, *You're released, but I want you to know that you have my blessing if you will continue to keep your attitude of being on your face before Me.* At that moment I said, "Lord, that's what you have taught me. I am willing to walk in it." Almost immediately I felt a full release of peace and freedom to move ahead.

Question: How did God answer and supply the new church building?

Henson: The church raised almost $300,000 in cash for the project. But that wasn't enough. I didn't understand how God was going to answer, but I knew I was to go ahead with the project. We began construction by asking for bids from contractors. This is where God answered prayer. Most of the bids came in at 50 percent or less than the price we expected to pay. Some contractors donated their labor and the church paid for the materials; some donated both. In all, we built a church building of $1.3 million and paid cash for it because God answered prayer. The church paid $625,000 against the $1.3 million dollar estimate of construction.

(Jerry Falwell and Elmer Towns spoke at the building dedication. They were amazed at testimony after testimony of various contractors telling how God spoke to them to do the construction at a vastly reduced price. Some of the contractors were nonbelievers and/or nonchurch men, but they did their work because they were impressed by God to do it. Most of these contractors were not from Lighthouse Baptist Church.)

Question: Why do you think God heard this prayer?

Henson: It's not the fast that God blesses, rather, God blesses the motive of the heart and the intentions of the heart. I think fasting is an outward tangible expression of what is happening in a man's heart. I think when a man fasts, he is saying, "I am serious enough about my need and desire to know God and seek God, that I am willing to sacrifice to get an answer from God." What may seem foolish in the eyes of the lost and some Christians really honors God. Your ability to sacrifice doesn't get results; God doesn't care what you sacrifice, He just wants to see your attitude in your fast.

Question: What other results have come from fasting?

Henson: In the last three years at Lighthouse, we've taken the month of March and committed it to prayer and fasting as a church body. We ask our people to commit to fast one day a week. We have developed prayer clocks. We have conducted extra prayer meetings, and this year we asked our people to commit to an additional week of fasting. We ask our people not to watch TV during their fast. We have had an unusual moving of the Spirit of God during this time. Where we would normally have 8 to 10 people pray to receive Christ in the course of the month, we had about 80 conversions during that month.

Question: What do you typically abstain from?

Henson: Everything but water. And during the 21-day fast, I only drank water. The Bible seems to teach this procedure; it is a way a person can have liberty in fasting. When I led our church to fast from TV for a week, which is an unusual kind of fast, I don't think that's contrary to the Bible. It's not exactly the kind of fast the Bible speaks about, but we've had some of the greatest spiritual results in our people's lives when they fast from TV. They not only learn a lot from it, but they also understand how often they are wasting their time, so there was a real spiritual impact upon their lives.

Question: What direction would you give a person who has never fasted? How would you get someone started?

Henson: Well, I would encourage them to start with Bible study so they understand the reasons for fasting and the motivation for fasting. Then I would encourage them to start small with just a one-day fast. Then I would encourage them, if they have good health, to try an extended fast. I would start with one day, and then at least try a three-day fast. And if they are able, try for more days than that.

The first time I ever had an extended fast my body really craved food. After you get into the third and fourth day, the body stops craving food. I have learned that the human body will cry out for something it really doesn't need to have. But you think you need it. After a period of time I learned that my body doesn't really need food as desperately as it cries out for food. And then I also find that the further I get into the fast, the more I sense God's presence. The communion I have with God deepens the further I get into a fast. So I would encourage someone to start with one day, but somewhere along the line, try to set aside time for an extended fast.

Question: Has fasting ever hurt you, or have you felt healthy because of a fast?

Henson: Every time I've fasted, I have always ended up healthier. Never has fasting hurt me.

⇒ TAKE-AWAYS ⇐

You can make a difference by fasting, because when you make a vow to seek God and pray, you can turn around circumstances. Just as Al Henson refused to submit to circumstances, so your fast can change your circumstances. Look at what he brought to his fast. You need a clear burden from God, a determination to know God and a rock-solid choice to hunger and thirst after God's answer while you fast from food. You will receive power to fast and pray after you make a decision to fast and pray.

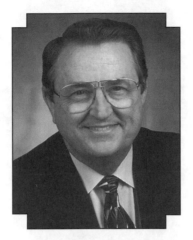

JIMMY DRAPER

President
The Sunday School Board
Southern Baptist Convention
Nashville, Tennessee

Jimmy Draper is the chief executive officer of the largest organization in the Southern Baptist Convention, which is the largest Protestant denomination in the world. Having a budget of more than $325 million, it is the largest publisher of religious books, Bibles, Sunday School literature and church material in the world. Draper has received several honorary doctorate degrees and has served as a minister of churches, mostly in Texas. He came to the Sunday School Board from pastoring First Baptist Church, Euless, Texas, which had an attendance of more than 3,000 weekly and an annual budget of $4 million. When he went to the church in 1975, it had 900 in attendance.

Draper has held most of the state and national offices in the Southern Baptist Convention, has had 22 books published and has traveled in more than 30 foreign nations to preach the gospel.

3

ASSURANCE OF GOD'S FORGIVENESS

Interview with

JIMMY DRAPER

Question: When did you first fast?

Draper: The first time I fasted, God came on me and I did not really have any choice but to fast, so my hunger was gone. I just knew I wanted to have a heart toward God because I had become mechanical and had lost the freshness in my walk with God. I was not doing anything bad; the church was great on the outside, but I knew inwardly I needed a closer walk with the Lord.

In 1969 when I was pastoring in Kansas City, I attended a Youth for Christ pastors' conference. Al Metzger presided, and Dave Boyer sang and gave his testimony. At the time of this conference, a real crisis was happening in my life.

I had been saved since I was five years old and I knew I was saved and had never doubted it. I never smoked, drank, never did anything typical of so many young people. That day as Dave spoke, however, God seemed to open up my heart and let me see how really wicked my natural man was. I started weeping. I left the conference because the last thing a preacher wants is for a crowd to see him crying. I drove back to my church and was still crying. I called the music minister, and tried to tell him what was happening, but all I could do was blubber. My staff knelt and prayed for me.

This incident caused me to begin to fast . . . I did not set out to fast, but I had no hunger . . . I was absolutely not hungry. I was so concerned with my own brokenness before God that I didn't eat for a week. I probably wouldn't have started eating again except we were planning a trip overseas. I felt I needed to have solid food for strength before going to the Holy Land.

I didn't choose to fast at this time. God just came on me in such a way that I could not eat.

Question: Were there other times God led you into fasting?

Draper: I'll be the first to say that I do not fast nearly as much as I should. But in a Bible conference in my church in 1976, God really convicted me. I had not been fasting any length of time, but I fasted for eight days at that time. Jerry Falwell was preaching at that conference when I was compelled to fast.

Question: Was there a specific purpose for which you were fasting?

Draper: I just wanted to hear from God! I felt that as a pastor I had gotten to the place where I was going through the motions. I was preaching and pastoring and doing everything I was supposed to do, but I needed a special touch from God in my own heart.

Question: What did God do for you?

Draper: It was an incredible time for me; it was probably one of the deepest spiritual experiences I had ever had. I am not generally an emotional person, but I was emotional during that time, and I was attending the Texas Baptist Convention. The director called for me to lead in prayer. It was a moment when God drew the attention of our convention toward a real brokenness before Him. It was a milestone in my own life of reconnecting me to that earlier experience. I have fasted since that time and I continue to do so when facing decisions from God.

Question: Tell us some of the personal disciplines you follow in fasting.

Draper: Well, I had not read any books on fasting at the time. When hunger would come during fasting, I would use that as an opportunity for Bible study, letting my hunger call me to God rather than leading me to food. When there were times that I would normally be eating food, I would spend that time in Bible study and prayer. To me the whole purpose of fasting is not to stop eating, but fasting is for times when there is such a hunger for God that eating is not important. To me fasting has come at times when my experience with God was so consuming that communion with God was more important than eating.

≩ TAKE-AWAYS ≩

Sometimes we fast and alter our diets to show we are sincere. After the fast, we meet God and He works in our lives. It was the opposite with Jimmy Draper. God met Draper in a pastors' meeting and he was so overwhelmed with God's presence that he did not eat for a week. The Hebrew word for fast comes from *tsome*, which implies distress—we are so distressed that we lose our appetites. Some fast to touch God; others fast after they have seen God.

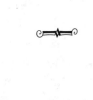

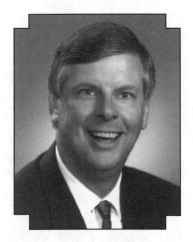

GENE MIMS

Vice President for Church Growth Group
The Sunday School Board
Southern Baptist Convention
Nashville, Tennessee

For almost 20 years, Gene Mims served as pastor of Southern Baptist churches in Texas, Virginia, Alabama and Tennessee. His calling has been to help churches evangelize the world, develop believers and assist churches to grow.

Under Mims's direction, the Church Growth Group of the Southern Baptist Convention has become a constant source of fresh and new services to help churches grow and expand their witness to the saving grace of Jesus Christ. Recently, Mims told a group of pastors, "The mandate of the Great Commission is our driving force, and our focus is meeting the needs of churches."

The responsibility of the Church Growth Group is to service Bible teaching, discipleship, family development and church leadership in the Southern Baptist Convention. Church music, administration, student ministries, church media library, architecture and recreation are also significant parts of the group's ministry.

Mims has earned master of divinity and doctor of ministry degrees from Southwestern Baptist Theological Seminary, Forth Worth, Texas, and has authored three books—*Thine Is the Kingdom, God's Call to a Corrupt Nation,* and *Kingdom Principles for Church Growth,* which is being used widely as "The Essential Guide for Church Growth" in Southern Baptist churches.

≝ 4 ≝

A NEW CALL FOR SERVICE

Interview with

GENE MIMS

Question: Gene, tell me about the first time you remember fasting.

Mims: The first time I remember fasting was as a student at Virginia Tech University. I was a sophomore and a member of the University InterVarsity Fellowship Campus group, and attending a Bible study, where the principle of fasting was discussed. Even though I had been a lifelong Southern Baptist, I had never thought about fasting. God put fasting on my heart, so one day I made a decision I would fast. Beginning the night before, I skipped dinner, and going through the next day, I concentrated on thinking about the Lord. I remember it like it was yesterday;

my communion with the Lord was something I had never experienced before. Fasting is something I have done and will do for the rest of my life. Even though I went about my college classes and studies, I didn't think about anything else. I thought about growing in the Lord, getting close to the Lord and deepening that relationship.

And it sure worked!

Question: Do you remember your time of prayer?

Mims: I got up in the morning and, instead of having breakfast, I prayed and read the Bible, as it has been a lifelong habit. I read a verse of Scripture and concentrated on Matthew 17:21, thinking not about me, but about God, until I had a release in my spirit to go to the next verse. What I thought would be about five minutes of study and prayer was probably in excess of a half hour or longer.

Question: How did you break your fast?

Mims: Interestingly enough, I wondered if you'd ask. I made a commitment that I would fast for one day and I was really set to eat the following day. I remembered feeling almost like I didn't want this to stop. I was frankly disappointed to have to eat and get back into my daily routine.

Question: Of all the times you have fasted, what would be the most significant project for which you have fasted?

Mims: There have been several, but probably the most significant time was recently when I was trying to make a determination whether to come and join Jimmy Draper at the Baptist Sunday School. I had been a pastor for 20 years—that is what I am. At the time, my wife and I were talking to a church's committee in Toronto, Canada, about the possibility of becoming its pastor. I didn't know what else to do so I took some time away with my father in North Carolina. I not only refrained from eating, but I also prayed and asked the Lord for His will and His direction. He answered me in clear and unmistakable terms. I was to go to the Baptist Sunday School Board.

Question: Give a step-by-step report about how God let you know about this decision.

Mims: I was talking to my father about my decision, and essentially I didn't know what to do: whether to pastor the church in Canada, or go to the Sunday School Board. I didn't have any experience in running a corporation. My father said something to the effect that the Lord would let me know. The next morning before 6:00 A.M. I had awakened and I was praying. I really felt the Lord was leading me . . . we were close . . . and He was about to speak to me, but I didn't know what He would say. I didn't know when He would give me an answer. I haven't told many people, but I had a vision of the Lord—in my mind, not actually. I had a pencil and a legal pad in my hand and the Lord told me to write down what I wanted to do. I went to write but couldn't. I handed the paper back to Him and said I wanted to do what He wanted me to do. Unmistakably, the Lord said I should go to the Baptist Sunday School Board. I never doubted that decision, even though there were some very difficult times ahead.

Question: What did you write while praying and fasting?

Mims: When I went back to look at some notes I had made, it basically said, "Lord, here are some things that I feel are critical for me to know." Of course, one of the things was where to go and serve. The other thing was if I went to the Sunday School Board, would it afford me the opportunity to become more like Christ and would I have a closer walk with the Lord as well? One of the reasons I put that down was that I couldn't understand how I could work as a denominational official in a corporation and still keep my pastoral heart and walk with Christ.

Question: Do you have a practical suggestion for someone else who is fasting?

Mims: First, you need to understand very clearly the nature of the fast. Why are you doing this? Are you doing this because of a burden? Is it a decision to purge a sin? Second, you need to understand the biblical range of what fasting is. Third, you need to determine the length of the fast. Some people think a fast is 40 days; some people don't. You need to know that a fast is for whatever period of time the Lord leads. Next, you must know the Lord is in this! You must feel good about what you are doing, not so much to direct God but so that God's heart and your heart come together. Then when you fast, block everything out and focus upon the Lord, not the issue for which you fast. Concentrate on His Word, think about God and then the Lord will either direct your path or He'll give you assurance that it is not right. In fasting you will draw closer to Him, which always gives you strength and assurance.

≩ TAKE-AWAYS ≩

When you face a life-changing decision, fast and pray for God's direction. God can first show you Himself and, second, guide you in the direction He would have you go.

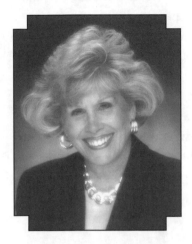

JANE A. HANSEN
International President
Aglow International
Edmonds, Washington

Jane Hansen serves as president/CEO of Aglow International, a worldwide outreach ministry that is influencing the lives of women in 137 nations. Some have said this is the largest international ministry to women.

She logs more than 100,000 miles annually throughout the United States and abroad to share a message of God's unique call to women in this significant decade. She has spoken before audiences on six continents. Her desire is for God's healing and restoration to reach into women's lives that they may embrace all God wills to do through them.

Keeping that goal in mind, Jane has searched the Scriptures for 20 years in order to understand God's plan to reconcile the relationship between men and women, a restoration that directly affects the family unit as God intended it to be—the basic expression of His love and relationship on earth. This message is found in her books *Fashioned for Intimacy* and *The Journey of a Woman*.

Jane serves in leadership roles in many organizations, including the Spiritual Warfare Network, the Advisory Council for the International Charismatic Consultation of World Evangelization, the Advisory Board for the Regent University School of Divinity, the International Board for the International Reconciliation Coalition, and the National Advisory Board for March for Jesus.

5

FREEING
A SON FROM
DRUGS

Interview with
JANE HANSEN

FAVORITE VERSE:
She looketh well to the ways of her household.
—*Proverbs 31:27*

Question: Tell me about the first time you fasted.

Hansen: I was facing a very difficult and painful situation in my family with a son who was a drug addict and an alcoholic. As a mother, I felt that I should somehow be able to make a difference in his life. As the burden for this son increased in my heart, I felt myself entering into a new kind of "laboring" for him. It was almost as though I were about to give birth to him again . . . not, of course in the physical sense, but in a spiritual sense. For me, that involved both praying and fasting.

Question: Will you please explain what you mean by giving birth to him in a spiritual sense and what part fasting played in that process?

Hansen: As women, we have been designed by God to give birth physically. But I believe He wants to use that very nature He has given us to bring some things to "birth" in the spiritual realm as well.

At times when the nation of Israel was in trouble, it was the women God called for. In Jeremiah 9:17 it states to "call for the mourning women." He was calling for skillful, wailing women to come to intercede for a people who were far from God so that they would repent. Why? Because death had crept into the nation . . . into the cities and streets and even into the homes. It was cutting off the children from life. It reads like today's newspaper. Death has crept into our nation and the nations of the world. It is our young people, our children, that have been most greatly affected by the increased violence. I believe in the day in which we live, with violence increasing in the earth, God is again calling for women to come to cry out to God on behalf of their families and the cities and nations of the world.

Because we know that biblical truth runs in a circular fashion, it gives us confidence that God wants to use His people today to "bring to birth" the things that are on His heart to do in this hour.

Question: What do you mean about truth running in a circular fashion?

Hansen: We often think prayer is about convincing God to do something we want. In reality, it is about entering into God's will, calling forth His kingdom to come in the earth, and this act is circular. The will, the plan and purpose of God begins in heaven, in God's heart. He is always looking for those on earth who have an ear to hear what He wants to do in the earth.

Those who hear will begin to carry this burden in the "womb of their spirit." When the fullness of time has come, there is a knowing in their heart, perhaps without even being able to articulate it clearly at first. They begin to press into God with greater fervency. They begin to pray and speak forth the heart of God in that situation. As His will and Word are accomplished, it flows back to heaven fulfilled as He purposed. It is what we say in the Lord's Prayer . . . Thy kingdom come, Thy will be done . . . in earth, . . . as it is in heaven!

Question: How did fasting play a part in this process?

Hansen: As the truth of God's Word began to impact my own heart, I felt a sense of urgency to give myself to Him fully that the victory He purposed might be accomplished. My full attention was drawn toward God. My "fast" was to include several aspects of my life. Rather than being out of the house, busily about many things that would distract, I was drawn, almost impelled, to fast my time and attention. I went out less, talked on the phone less, watched TV less, gave myself to the reading of the Word and prayer more. It was a most fulfilling season. Again, not unlike a mother preparing for the imminent birth of a new child.

Question: Did your fast include food as well?

Hansen: In part, it did. Because I have a problem with blood sugar levels, I was not able to go long periods of time without food. I eliminated certain foods, or meals, but I have found that it is the attitude of heart and the coming aside unto Him that God is most after.

Question: What was the attitude of your heart at this time?

Hansen: It was an attitude of total victory. Somehow my heart had been quickened by the reading of the Word and I just knew that this was a battle for the soul of my son and God's enemy would not win. My part was to proclaim God's Word into this situation. I decided to intercede and not quit until the answer had come. Today, my son is a man who walks with the Lord.

Question: What are the greatest things for which you have fasted?

Hansen: First was the situation with my son. I believe God broke his addiction to drugs and alcohol through prayer and fasting.

Another incident is related to my marriage. Both my husband and I were raised in pastors' homes. At this point in our lives, my husband had not yet come to a place of a personal relationship with Christ. There were several points of stress and difficulty in our marriage. I began to fast and pray for this situation as well as the situation with my son.

I have seen the walls my husband had placed around himself come down. His heart, that was once so closed, has opened to God and to me. Today, he serves as an elder in our church. He is a loving, caring husband and father.

I see the activity of the Proverbs 31 woman not only as physical, but spiritual. She looks well to the ways of her household. That word "looks" is similar to the word in Ezekiel for "watchman." She is like a watchman in her home. God will use her to bring forth His heart, will and purpose in her family. Fasting will play a part in that.

⊰ TAKE-AWAYS ⊱

You can continually fast and pray for a family member who is in bondage or addiction and God will answer your prayer. Those who physically can't fast can enter the spirit of fasting to get results.

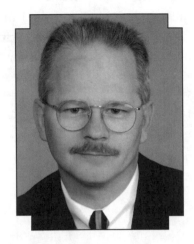

DAVID EARLEY

Senior Pastor, New Life Community Baptist Church
Gahanna (Greater Columbus), Ohio

Dave Earley is senior pastor of New Life Community Baptist Church, Gahanna, Ohio. He founded the church along with a team of four graduates from Liberty University in 1985. Since then, the church has grown from 12 to an average weekly attendance of more than 900 and a staff of 15. The present facilities are valued at more than $4 million, including a 1,000-seat multiuse auditorium.

Prior to planting New Life, Dave was Director of Discipleship for students at Liberty University. He has also served as president of a church-planting organization, Change a Nation, Inc. He has received awards for preaching, church planting and the Eagle award as Alumnus of the Year from Liberty University. Dave graduated from Liberty University in 1981 (summa cum laude) with a B.S. in pastoral counseling, earned his M.Div. from Liberty Baptist Theological Seminary (magna cum laude) in 1985 and was awarded the doctor of ministry degree by Liberty in 1998.

Dave has authored several church-growth resources, including *How to Move Believers from Membership to Maturity to Ministry: A Progressive Discipleship Program*; *Prime Time: A Daily Guide for Spending Time with God*; and *Together Everyone Accomplishes More: A Stewardship Plan for Multiplying Your Ministry.*

6

PLANTING A NEW CHURCH

Interview with

DAVID EARLEY

Question: How did you first learn about fasting?

Earley: A few days before I first came to Liberty in 1977, a friend of mine encouraged me to spend a few days fasting and praying with him. We went to Long's Retreat, which is a campground about 40 minutes from my home in Chillicothe, Ohio. During that time, God spoke more clearly than He ever had previously.

Question: What did you learn about fasting at Liberty?

Earley: When I first got to Liberty, J. O. Grooms taught us personal evangelism, and also how to fast. I began to fast one day, every week, on Tuesdays. I probably began to fast my freshman year, about my second or third week at college. For me it was a great spiritual benefit, even though I was on the wrestling team. We had three-hour, very demanding practices on Tuesdays, the day of my fast. It was a great faith-building event to learn that God would give me physical energy to do well in practice even though I would go without food.

Question: When did you actually begin your fast?

Earley: I would eat dinner on Monday night, then eat dinner again on Tuesday night. I fasted breakfast and lunch.

Question: What happened during those fasts?

Earley: I think I am still seeing God answering prayers from what happened during those times. My prayer time was from 12 to 1 every day in the operating room of an old hospital that was our dorm.

Question: Describe the call to church planting and what role fasting played in that endeavor.

Earley: After 1979, I was traveling on the Jesus First Evangelistic Team with Harold Vaughn and other students. We ministered in approximately 70 churches in about 70 days. We visited mostly new church plants. During that time I was reading about the call of God in John R. Rice's life. God then called me to plant a new church. I began to pray every day for a town, a team and a time to go do it. I especially prayed for these three things on the day set aside for fasting. In 1981, God gave me my first teammate, Cathy, my wife. In December 1981, four men made commitments to be a part of the team: Rod Dempsey, Steve Benninger, Brian Robertson and Chris Brown. We all went to Greater Columbus, Ohio, four years later to begin a church. While we were students, we fasted for the church God put upon our hearts.

Every week as I fasted, the picture of the new church came into focus. I felt God calling me to the Midwest . . . Columbus, Ohio, . . . then to a specific suburb in Columbus. And by 1983, we knew the town, we had the team and we were set to go in 1985.

Question: How long were you fasting for the location of your church plant?

Earley: About six years before we started the church. I was still fasting for a church mainly one day a week.

Question: What is the greatest answer you have ever had as far as fasting and prayers are concerned?

Earley: Probably every good thing in my life has been the result of fasting and praying. One of the biggest answers was in 1992. Our church was out of educational space. We had moved into a building but we were not in the position financially to build additional space. Every winter we had set aside a week or a month for prayer and fasting as a church.

In 1992, we challenged our people to eight great days of fasting. I was one of the people fasting all those eight days. On the last day of our fast, I got a call from a businessman who is not a member of our church. He knew we needed more education space. He told me that God told him to give us $70,000. He wanted to know if I would take it. I told him I would. Within a few weeks after that we were able to add six classrooms and continue to grow as a church. God gave us $70,000 after eight great days of prayer and fasting. That was in February 1992; we dedicated the new facility by the end of May 1992.

Question: What has God done for your personal worship of Him through fasting?

Earley: Individually, some of my sweetest times with God have been as a result of fasting and worship. In the early days of our church, I was the only full-time staff person and had the office building to myself. On several occasions after a two- or three-day fast, I had the privilege of experiencing a level of personal commitment that was incredible. The presence of God was so real that it was as though time stopped. The light of His glory seemed tangible. I felt indescribable love and cleansing. Jesus was so precious that no other thoughts entered my mind. I was wonderfully lost in His presence.

Question: When you are getting ready to lead a group of people into fasting, how do you do it?

Earley: When I want to lead people into fasting, I usually teach a sermon or a series of sermons about spiritual and practical guidelines of fasting. I also recommend books such as *Fasting for Spiritual Breakthrough* by Elmer Towns, *God's Chosen Fast* by Arthur Wallis and the book by Bill Bright, *The Coming Revival.* I also make available tapes of sermons I have preached in the past on fasting. This past winter, we had a hundred people commit to fasting one day a week for 10 weeks. And to prepare them, we mailed them information and assigned them a prayer partner. On Sunday nights I taught an eight-week series on fasting. We were also able to make available the video seminar by Elmer Towns, *Fasting for Spiritual Breakthrough.*

Question: What would be the typical events you would do in a day of fasting?

Earley: I like to fast on Mondays. Usually I eat a light dinner early on Sunday evenings. Then after church I don't watch television. On Monday I get up for my regular time of journaling, prayer and Bible reading. During the day I work as usual. I drink an eight-ounce bottle of juice and dilute it with water. When I finish that, I drink several glasses of distilled water. I fast until about three o'clock on Monday. I like to block out extra time over the breakfast hour or after the lunch time for extra prayer. About three o'clock, I eat a couple of crackers. On Monday evening I eat a normal dinner. About every other month I go to a private retreat or hotel and spend the whole day in fasting and praying. Once a year I like to get away somewhere to spend about three days fasting and praying.

Question: Who goes with you?

Earley: Usually, I go alone. On a couple of occasions I have taken a staff member.

Question: You had some lingering physical problems. Did fasting cause those problems or interrupt your daily requirements?

Earley: In August 1991, I got a type of flu called Epstein-Barr virus, which is commonly called "chronic fatigue syndrome." Basically, I got the flu that would not go away. I lost 18 pounds in three weeks. I began to experience severe joint pain. Eventually, it began to affect most areas of my life. For a couple of years, on the recommendations of the doctors, I was not allowed to fast. In the past two years, they have started allowing me to get back to fasting one day a week or more. As a result, my health has improved significantly. A couple of times I went on a three-day fast under the directions of doctors, primarily for the benefit of detoxing my system. I noticed when I started fasting regularly again, my health continued to improve.

Question: What directions would you give to those who have never fasted; how would you get them started?

Earley: I encourage people to start small. Usually fast one meal the first time. Maybe two meals for the second time and then a whole 24 hours. Then a two- or three-day fast. I encourage them to drink a lot of juice or water, and to limit their physical activity, and I encourage them to plan their fast at times when they can spend extra time with God. Recently, I have begun to encourage people to have a prayer partner praying for them on their fast day. Before going on an extended fast, they probably need to get a doctor's approval. It is a good idea to tell friends and family when going on a long fast so they understand why meals are being missed. They can also pray for the person fasting. People should expect that they will not feel well physically while fasting and might not feel well spiritually either while fasting. But the results are worth it. Sometimes people notice greater demonic attacks when they are fasting. It means they are making an impact for God's kingdom.

This winter, I felt God lead me to get our entire city to fast and pray. We got 15 churches to work together to distribute a copy of the *Jesus* video, free to every home in our city. Several people from various churches met on Mondays for an hour and a half at lunch. We met at a different church every week to pray for revival in our city and to pray for the distribution of the *Jesus* video. As a result, we had one of the most successful citywide efforts Campus Crusade has ever had. We distributed 6,300 copies of the *Jesus* video in two hours. During the course of a few weeks, the number went up to 8,000 copies of the video, and more than 600 people told us they had made decisions for Christ.

≩ TAKE-AWAYS ≨

You should try to make fasting a regular discipline in your life by planning to fast on a weekly or monthly routine. You should also try to plan special events to pray for longer times, or go to a special place for prayer and fasting.

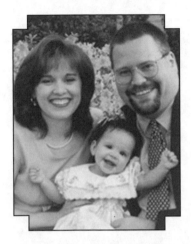

TROY TEMPLE

Instructor, Center for Youth Ministries
Liberty University, Lynchburg, Virginia

Troy Temple is an instructor in the Department of Church Ministries at Liberty University, Lynchburg, Virginia. He also serves as the director of Youth Ministry Services for the Center for Youth Ministry at Liberty, and he supervises the annual Harvesttime House of Death called ScareMare, attended by approximately 20,000 people each year. Last year more than 3,000 decisions for Christ were made.

He has served as a youth pastor and is committed to local church ministry. He currently serves in the Middle School Department at Thomas Road Baptist Church, Lynchburg, Virginia, and is also a frequent camp and youth seminar speaker.

Troy and his wife, Karla, have been married for seven years. They have a daughter, Madeleine, and make their home in Lynchburg, Virginia.

7

A BABY GIRL
FOR A CHILDLESS
COUPLE

Interview with

TROY TEMPLE

FAVORITE VERSE ABOUT FASTING:

So we fasted and petitioned our God about this,
and he answered our prayer.
—*Ezra 8:23, NIV*

Question: When did you fast?

Temple: I fasted from the beginning of February through the middle of March in 1997. It was a 40-day fast . . . the Lord led me into it primarily for spiritual renewal . . . for a new financial discipline in my personal finances . . . and also for a family . . . a child. My wife and I had been infertile for six years.

Question: Describe the financial aspects of your fast.

Temple: After the fast was over, my wife and I actually began living on a budget. We had not been disciplined before this. As a result of the fast, we were able to give more, and since that time we have seen our giving increase. We got to the point where we were not necessarily wondering where the money was coming from, as we were before the fast.

Question: How long have you been married?

Temple: At the time of the fast we had been married five and a half years.

Question: How serious were your financial troubles?

Temple: We were not in deep financial trouble, but we were to the point where it was paycheck to paycheck. Nothing left over. After payday came, and for two weeks, there was no spending money. There was no money for an occasional lunch out, no money for any incidentals or emergencies that came up . . . it was very insecure as far as knowing that things would be provided for.

Question: How did God change you?

Temple: Through the fast, God began to simplify my spiritual life by focusing on Him and my becoming more like Him. God focused my relationship with Him. Two areas came out of that, . . . one was something I wasn't even praying about: my physical health and my personal diet so I could stay healthy for a long time to care for my family. Second, financially, God convicted me about my misuse of funds, not unethical misuse of funds, but purchasing things on the spur of the moment . . . purchasing things I didn't really need. There was a lack of discipline in regard to financial matters. In fasting, God convicted me to be the spiritual leader in our home, carrying it through all areas: financially, physically for the health of my family, and leading them in all areas.

Question: Are you on a budget now?

Temple: We're on a budget now. We've been on it for about a year and a half. In fact, I am planning this very next week . . . in December. . . before Christmas week to meet with our financial counselor. We'll revisit the budget now that we have a little girl, and set up a new budget to allow for retirement and to fin-ish paying off consumer debt we got into.

Question: Tell me about your family.

Temple: Karla and I were married in 1991. Within the first year, after prayer, we tried to begin our family. At that time, we conceived twice in our second year of marriage. Both times we lost the children—Jordan was the first child to miscarry and Taylor our second child, in late 1992. From that time on we were never able to conceive. We consulted specialists, and spent a lot of income trying to diagnose two years of unexplained infertili-ty. No problem was pinpointed.

About a year ago my wife spoke with Ruth Towns, director of a local adoption agency our church supported. It is also where we ended up getting our little girl. Karla asked questions, and Ruth encouraged her to fill out the application and come in to talk with her, which we did. At that time, we were very encour-aged about the possibilities . . . but still really troubled by the unexplained infertility . . . we weren't completely resolved with that whole issue. We didn't know why God had done what He had done.

A month later, I sat on an ordination council for a friend of mine in North Carolina. He had been on a 40-day fast, and ended it the very evening they had the ordination ceremony. As I was driv-ing home by myself, I was convicted in several areas. One had to do with my physical health and financial discipline. I literally wrestled with God in the three-hour drive. I sang hymns and the Holy Spirit was my copilot, convicting me about these areas of my life.

The Holy Spirit asked me several questions. What would I be willing to do to influence my family for a long time? Would I be willing to become a financial steward of the resources God had given me? What would I be willing to do to have integrity and be able to impact people's lives through giving? The questions came in the car, "Are you willing to meet with Me and fast for 40 days?"

After about two hours of wrestling with God, I just said,

"Father, I will do whatever it takes to be the man in my home that you need me to be, financially, physically and spiritually for my wife, for my family and for the future."

Question: What commitment did you make?

Temple: I committed to do an actual fast. My friend had done a water-only diet. At the time, I didn't have a lot of information about different types of fasts. I learned more when I talked to Elmer Towns about the different kinds of fasts and their purposes. I began with juice and water only, and stuck to it. That was my original commitment. No solid food . . . no warm food . . . no soup. Only juice and water. I became very fond of cranapple juice, and still am. I actually went out and purchased a juicer and started juicing vegetables and fruits, and am still very much sold on the physical enrichment and value of that discipline and practice.

Question: Describe your prayer time during your fast.

Temple: I had a list of people in my Day-Timer for whom I would pray every day—first, personal or spiritual renewal; second, financial discipline; and third, a child for my wife and me. I was praying for God to multiply our family.

Question: How did God answer?

Temple: In September 1997, my wife and I had submitted an application to the agency we had previously contacted. (Not the agency where Ruth Towns was located.) They changed their fee structure . . . and it was very disappointing because the fee structure went from something we could manage to something that was insurmountable in cost. We decided to put it on hold. Ruth Towns came to my wife's office in the church and questioned her about why we hadn't completed an application with the agency where she was director. We then met with her, and she explained that a hard-to-place child would require the same adoption fees we were able to pay at the other agency before they raised their fees. We had already prayed about taking a hard-to-place child, so we agreed right then and there . . . and we even prayed with

Ruth . . . the Lord led us right to that point. It was a decision that didn't take much effort to make. God was in it.

At the very time we were talking with Ruth Towns, a birth mother was being interviewed in another office in the same building. We didn't meet because it is a confidential adoption. A social worker was meeting with the birth mother and came into Ruth's office and explained that this mother had seen the photo albums of the parents and the families that were willing to adopt hard-to-place children. The birth mother didn't choose any of them.

The social worker wanted to know if we were interested in giving her a biographical sketch and a photograph to show this birth mother the next Tuesday. We spent the whole weekend redoing a complete photo album, birth letters to the mother—I wrote one, my wife wrote one—we did an update, a whole biographical sketch. The very next Tuesday the birth mother saw our album. They didn't tell us she was interested in us. This agency sometimes will not tell details because some birth mothers change their minds.

On Wednesday while I was teaching a class, a student came and said, "Mr. Temple, do you have any kids?"

I replied, "No, Jenna, why do you ask?"

She said, "I don't know but God has laid it upon my heart to tell you that you're going to be a dad soon."

The agency got a call from the birth mother that day, saying we were the only family she could picture with her little girl . . . Troy and Karla are to be her parents. Within eight to nine weeks we had our daughter. She is beautiful and she fits our family and even looks like me . . . dark hair and brown eyes. Her name is Madeleine.

What is incredible is the timing. God touched me . . . driving down the road and I made a commitment to a 40-day fast. Madeleine's birth mother conceived her during the middle of my 40-day fast. The providence of God brought me to tears. I was distraught, emotionally at my wit's end, and also physically at my weakest, but at that time God had already begun to prepare a little girl for my wife and me. The whole power and magnitude of God's sovereignty was overwhelming.

That 40-day fast changed my life. I spent time begging and laying myself out before God asking to become a father . . . and my wife to become a mother . . . God didn't have to do that . . . it wasn't a negotiated bargain . . . I didn't trade food for God to give us a child . . . I humbled myself and didn't know how He was going to do it . . . and even through September when we were at our wit's end, little did I know that when I actually gave up something . . . that I didn't think I could afford to give up . . . through that 40-day fast, God began answering a six-year-long prayer of the battle with infertility. We now have Madeleine Paige, an answer to prayer.

≡ TAKE-AWAYS ≧

When we fast and pray for answers from God, He doesn't always answer the way we think He will answer. God has more than one way to answer our prayers. God gave a child to a couple through adoption rather than through conception. We must be patient when fasting for results; it may take nine months or longer to get results.

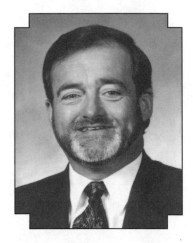

LARRY S. BOAN

Associate Pastor
Central Assembly of God
Vero Beach, Florida

Larry Boan is the associate pastor of Central Assembly of God in Vero Beach, Florida, where he has served for 17 years. He has felt God's call to a supportive position in a local church and has been both a youth pastor and associate pastor in Rock Hill, South Carolina, where he was born.

8

SALVATION
OF A DAD

Interview with
LARRY BOAN

FAVORITE VERSE ABOUT FASTING:

"I have been crucified with Christ; it is no longer I who
live, but Christ lives in me; and the life which I now live
in the flesh I live by faith in the Son of God, who
loved me and gave Himself for me."
—*Galatians 2:20, NKJV*

Question: Tell me how you began fasting for your dad.

Boan: Two years ago in January (1995) I was helping my wife
around the house, and just thinking about my dad. We had just
seen him and found out he had cancer. My dad was not a believer and had never attended church on a regular basis all of my life.
Only occasionally did he attend church, such as a funeral or
when I was visiting would he go to church. As I was helping my

wife . . . I felt the Lord speaking to me, asking, "Are you willing to fast for your dad?"

I said, "Yes, Sir, I am."

At that point I felt the Lord wanted me to fast for 40 days for my dad's salvation. So I began a 40-day fast. The twentieth day of the fast, I was visiting him in Rock Hill, South Carolina, where he lives. That day, when we were visiting and talking, I felt a little shifting in his attitude toward Christ. Later that evening, I asked Dad if I could pray for him.

He said, "Son, come back in about an hour and I will let you pray for me." He was pretty much bedridden, confined to his bed area.

Question: What was your dad's medical problem?

Boan: He had cancer, which was terminal.

Question: How did you feel about his response?

Boan: He had never said before that I could pray for him. He used to say, "Quit praying for me. Every time you pray for me, I get worse." This time he said, "Come back in an hour and I will let you pray for me." I was ecstatic about his answer. So I walked out to tell my wife and my mom.

I walked around the block, praying, "God, let me tell him about salvation, and let him respond. Give me Your favor in this regard."

When I went back and asked him if I could pray for him, he said, "Yes." I began to pray for him and I just asked the Lord to touch him and be with him. At that moment, I felt the Lord tell me that my father had already prayed.

When I finished praying, I asked Dad, "Have you already prayed?"

He said, "Yes."

I asked, "When did you pray?"

He responded, "A little while ago."

I said, "What did you pray?"

He said, "I asked God to accept me."

At that point he gave his heart to the Lord. Two weeks and

four days later, my dad died. On the fortieth day of my fast, we had his funeral. I was still fasting. I wanted to honor my commitment to fast for 40 days. The timing was something profound that the Lord did in my life.

Question: What kind of fast was this? Did you drink juice?

Boan: I drank juices and occasionally I had tomato soup. Most of the time it was juices but not total absence of food. It was mainly juices.

⇥ TAKE-AWAYS ⇤

God may put a burden upon you to fast because
He wants you to become involved in His work.
Sometimes we want a loved one converted, and we
just pray about it. Perhaps the Lord tests our sincerity
to see if we would fast for someone's conversion.

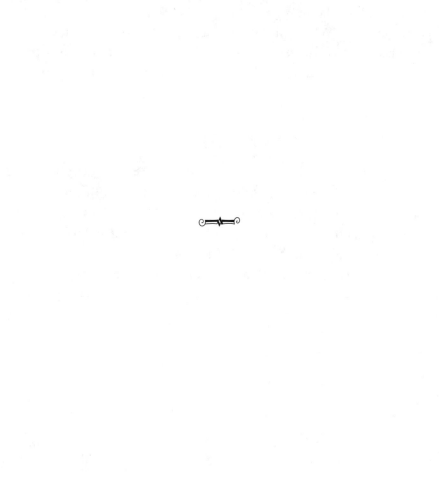

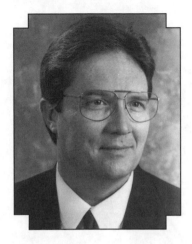

MICHAEL WOMACK

Pastor, Calvary Baptist Church
Erwin, Tennessee

Mike left the Agape Players in the summer of 1971 to attend Bible college in his hometown of Miami, Florida. Later he served as youth and music director in a Baptist church in Hialeah, Florida, before moving to Texas to attend Dallas Theological Seminary where he earned the Th.M. degree in 1982. After graduation, Mike and his wife, Claudia, moved to Tennessee where he continues to serve as senior pastor at Calvary Baptist Church in Erwin, Tennessee. Mike has also earned a D.Min. from Mid-America Baptist Theological Seminary in Memphis.

⊰ 9 ⊱

BUYING A BUS
FOR A
MUSICAL TEAM

Interview with
MICHAEL WOMACK

FAVORITE VERSE ABOUT FASTING:

David therefore besought God for the child; and David
fasted, and went in, and lay all night upon the earth.
—2 *Samuel 12:16*

Question: What did God do through fasting?

Womack: After coming to the Lord in early 1970, I had the
opportunity to travel with a group of about 25 other college-age
young people, doing music and drama evangelism across the
United States and Canada. We had purchased an old bus with the
proceeds of selling some 10,000 dozen Krispy Kreme donuts. I
recall major problems with the bus in almost every state. That
fall it seemed the bus was on its last legs, and we believed we

must have more reliable transportation. We were in Ohio at the time and staying in private homes in the Dayton area. After considerable thought, we agreed together to enter a time of fasting for a newer bus.

Most of us were young Christians and few of us had any actual experience with fasting. We agreed to an extended fast of a 30- to 40-day duration and felt it would be best if we allowed ourselves one glass of orange juice each morning and a glass of water later in the day. During our praying we also felt that God would be pleased to allow us to let our need be known to people we had met along the way.

Our phone bill became quite large, but God heard our prayers and blessed our calls by allowing us to receive enough money for us to purchase a used Greyhound Bus from a place in Chicago. The last day of our fast was the day before Thanksgiving, and the good people of Landmark Baptist Temple in Cincinnati let us break our fast in their fellowship hall by feeding us a large Thanksgiving Day banquet. We ate to our hearts' content, and not one of us became ill. Today, I would never recommend such a hearty meal to break a fast, but we were young and it was so very good.

Question: How did Landmark Baptist know of your need?

Womack: While staying in the Dayton area, we were able to sing and perform our evangelistic drama in many churches. Landmark was one of those places, and the people there were so very gracious. Did I tell you that the women of the church actually prepared the banquet for us?

Question: Did your group have a name?

Womack: We were called the Agape Players, and were comprised mostly of young adults from the Miami, Florida, area. In retrospect, I guess you could say we were sort of a noncharismatic addition to the Jesus People movement of the early 1970s. Rocky and Alice Adkins were the directors, and it was their vision as local church volunteers that brought the group together. As we traveled, people would join the group. One man was saved on a Sunday and left with us the following Tuesday. It was a wonderful group of zealous believers. We actually began with a borrowed Christian school bus before we bought the old 1948 Arrow Coach bus that got us as far as Ohio.

≩ TAKE-AWAYS ≧

God honors the fast of people who are not sure how to do it, but God answers when they look to God by faith and follow what they know the Bible teaches. They didn't just fast, however; it was accomplished by faith and works. They sold donuts to buy the first bus and made telephone calls to solicit money to purchase the second bus.

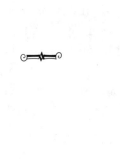

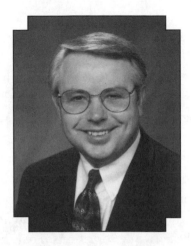

DAVID RHODENHIZER
Pastor, Calvary Road Baptist Church
Alexandria, Virginia

Pastor Rhodenhizer accepted Jesus as his personal Lord and Savior at Thomas Road Baptist Church under the ministry of Jerry Falwell on August 28, 1966. At the age of 16, Dave surrendered to the Lord's call to preach, but Falwell was not sure of his usefulness in ministry because David stuttered. Regardless of David's inability to understand why God would call him to preach despite his speech impediment, he has never doubted the call. As David looks back on those early days of his Christian journey, he realizes now that what he may have considered as one of the worst things in his life (the speech problem) was in reality one of the best things God could ever have done for him.

When God called David to preach, he was not healed immediately, nor was he healed sensationally. He testifies that his healing came gradually. Every time he tried to preach, God helped him and eventually more and more of the impediment was lifted. He testified, "I preached every opportunity I had, but people did not give me many opportunities." To that he adds with hindsight, "People did not try to dissuade me from preaching; I think they just did not encourage me because they did not want me to do something that would lead to disappointment."

David remembers not hesitating to tell others that God had called him to preach. "Regardless of whether people believed me or not, I wanted to obey God rather than man. I constantly asked God to remove my impediment."

Consider these two observations: First, he announced in faith that he was called to preach (a statement that showed confidence in God's ability to heal him). A second step of faith was when he attempted to preach without the ability (demonstrating that his desire to preach was not of the flesh).

David graduated from Liberty in 1974 with a B.S. degree and was later awarded the doctor of divinity degree. He planted Open Door Baptist Church in 1977 and later merged with Calvary Road Baptist Church. Today, the church averages almost 1,000 in attendance, has more than $5 million in assets and is a spiritual influence on the Greater Washington, D.C., community.

10

BREAKING STUTTERING

Interview with

DAVID RHODENHIZER

FAVORITE VERSE ABOUT FASTING:

If ye abide in me, and my words abide in you, ye shall
ask what ye will, and it shall be done unto you.

—*John 15:7*

Question: What was one of your greatest answers to prayer?

Rhodenhizer: Obviously, the greatest answer had to do with
God healing me so I could minister. There are several versions of
how God healed me, but let me tell you the events in sequence
so you can understand that in answer to prayer and fasting God
progressively healed me.

Several months before the summer of 1968, God had begun to
stir my heart concerning full-time Christian service. In May 1968,
I yielded my heart, and committed my life to go into the ministry to be a preacher of the gospel. This was nothing unusual. I

was not the first to be called into ministry, nor would I be the last. But, in a way, my situation was unique because I had a speech impediment. I had great difficulty communicating. I stuttered—some call it stammering. Although I could be reasonably understood, it would take me longer to communicate.

When my pastor, Dr. Jerry Falwell, heard that I had surrendered my life to preach the gospel, he thought I had somehow misread the leading of the Lord. After all, if I could not communicate reasonably well, how could I preach?

When I was a junior in high school, I met with a man from the Virginia Board of Vocational Rehabilitation. During my time with him, he told me that, essentially, because of my speech impediment, I was being offered a scholarship to attend either the University of Virginia or Virginia Polytechnic Institute. Basically, all that I would need would be my parents' signatures. Looking back, I suppose those schools offered good speech therapy courses and I assumed this was the reason the offer was being made. But not long before this meeting, God had called me to preach. I had one question for this gentleman. Could they help me through a Christian school? He kindly shared with me that they could not and so my answer was very simple. God would put me through a Christian school.

Many probably would think I was making a mistake, but I knew in my heart that I was doing exactly what God had told me. Although I had difficulty speaking, I knew God would take care of my speech impediment. My responsibility was to obey Him and to be faithful to His call.

During those early and eager days of my life, I had a desire to preach, but I couldn't find a preaching opportunity. I believe no one was being unkind, but I think some may have thought it would be a mistake to encourage me to do something that would cause me or them embarrassment. Eventually, I was asked to speak in an adult Sunday School class. I believe the teacher was Ed Martin. I will always be grateful for his confidence in me.

Next, an opportunity to teach a Sunday School class at Thomas Road Baptist Church came my way. R. C. Worley and I led the class. To this day, I'm not sure whether the class was given to me or to Brother Worley. I taught and he prayed and served as bouncer in this class of 13-year-old boys. I loved it! This growing, exciting Sunday School class was a great blessing and encouragement to me.

When I was a senior at E. C. Glass High School, the Lord impressed on me to start a Bible club in the public school. I remember going to the principal's office to seek his permission to begin the club. As we talked, he was not only pleased and supportive, but he also related to me that he had attended a Christian college. He gave me permission. Once a week on Friday I met with a few students for Bible study and prayer before classes began. This was a great step of faith as I watched God orchestrate the details.

As a young man, I can remember the concern, even the hurt, of not understanding why I would be called to preach and not be able to speak very well. Opportunities to speak and preach were slow to come my way because of my problem. People were never cruel, but, at the same time, I believe they thought they were sparing my feelings by not asking me to speak.

To this day, I have never doubted God's call to preach the gospel. As a teenager, though, I can remember kneeling beside my bed, broken, at times even weeping, because I did not understand why God would call me to preach when I could not talk. Now, as I look back on it, what I thought was the worst thing in my life—my speech impediment—had motivated me to completely rely upon the Lord's strength and trust Him to do in my life what only He could do. I had no natural talents or abilities. Whatever God was going to do with my life, He would have to do. You see, true faith is not praying, "Lord, if you will heal me, I will preach." For me, true faith was saying, "Lord, I will preach regardless of any healing."

During those early days of my Christian life and call to ministry, I cultivated a dependence and reliance upon God, and God alone, who would be my strength all the days of my life and ministry. God knew exactly what He was doing when He gave me that speech impediment. Now, every time I stand to preach God's Word, it is a testimony to the fact that in our weakness, He is strong. Everything that has taken place in my life in these past 30 years is an absolute credit to the faithfulness and power of the Lord Jesus Christ. I love Him more now than ever!

As I moved out of my teens and into my early 20s, opportunities began to come. God began to lift the speech impediment and I began to speak better and better. I believe God healed me, not instantly as I had prayed many times, but God healed me slowly so my faith would grow as He helped me speak without stuttering. To this day, I still have some of that speech impediment. I believe the Lord left it there as a reminder to me of His grace and strength. I believe that if I were to ever step out of His will for my life, the speech impediment would return. When I stand in the pulpit, God gives me the liberty to preach His Word with a clear voice. To God be all the glory for the great things He hath done!

Question: What experience of fasting do you recall?

Rhodenhizer: Well, I wouldn't consider myself an expert on fasting, but I do recall one event. In 1989, our church was going to have J. Harold Smith come to speak for a crusade. I was reading the devotional *Our Daily Bread*, which had a text on fasting. I just felt led to fast. I decided that I would fast for one day a week, indefinitely. For about two and a half years I selected one day every week to fast. I believe that the only exceptions were during vacation time with my family.

Question: Did you eat or drink?

Rhodenhizer: I would have either coffee or juice. No food!

Question: Were there other times of prayer and fasting in the life of the church?

Rhodenhizer: I called the church to pray and fast for 40 days before Easter in 1996. Of course, everyone was encouraged to pray every day. In addition, I challenged everyone to fast one day a week during this time. The church had invited the evangelist Tim Lee as the special speaker. We had an all-time-high attendance day of 2,051 people.

Question: What conversions happened on that day?

Rhodenhizer: It was magnificent! I think more than 58 people prayed to receive Christ.

Question: How did you lead the people into fasting for 40 days?

Rhodenhizer: I preached sermons on fasting as part of the preparation to educate them about just exactly what fasting is. Fasting is abstaining from food for the purpose of sharing with the Lord our desire for Him to do something in our lives. That's the primary purpose of fasting, and whatever side results may happen are good, but spiritual fasting is to abstain from food for God to be glorified.

Question: What other answers have come because of prayer?

Rhodenhizer: My daughter Melodie had *patent ductus*, a heart defect. A specialist at Georgetown University Hospital was treating her. We were just starting the church . . . there were a lot of pressures . . . and one morning as I had my devotions, I read from John 15:7, "If ye abide in me, and my words abide in you, ye shall ask what ye will, and it shall be done unto you."

I told the Lord that if He didn't do something special for me that day I would just as soon die. I asked the Lord to heal my little girl. We went to the hospital for the first procedure, which was a cardiac catheterization. We were briefed about what could happen. She would possibly need heart surgery, and she could have brain damage. You can't imagine what that did to my wife, Linda, and me. The doctor came back to the hospital room after the procedure, scratching his head.

He said, "I just don't understand it, it's gone! It had shown up on the X rays, but it is gone."

The Lord answered prayer and healed her. That answer to prayer did something for our new church. That new church learned that God really does answer prayer.

＃ TAKE-AWAYS ＃

You may not get a great answer the first time you fast, or the second time or even after repeated fasting. Sometimes you may have to fast for years before God answers your prayer. Some exercise great faith for a sudden miraculous healing, but you may have to exercise even greater faith over a longer period of time for God to intervene and answer your prayer. And even when you are waiting for God's answer, God may want you to begin serving Him with what you have (i.e., just as David Rhodenhizer began preaching before he was entirely healed). Then you may have to keep trusting God for the rest of your life, just as Rhodenhizer does because he believes his stuttering would return if he turned his back on God.

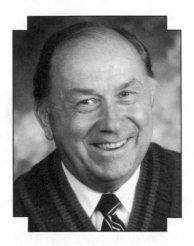

ELMER TOWNS
Dean, School of Religion
Liberty University, Lynchburg, Virginia

Elmer Towns is cofounder of Liberty University, along with Jerry Falwell, coming to Lynchburg, Virginia, in 1971 to begin the college as an extension of Thomas Road Baptist Church. He was the only full-time professor in its first year, teaching Bible, evangelism and theology. Because he prefers to teach, he chose not to be president, but rather to teach a full class schedule. When he turned 65 in 1997, he took on a threefold goal: to keep on learning, to keep on teaching what he learns and to keep on writing what he teaches.

Towns has written approximately 70 books, a great number by human comparison. When asked why so many, he says, "Every time I learn something new, like a teacher writing a complete lesson plan, I want to go a step further.

I want to write it into a book, i.e., into a complete package so others can read it and learn the things I've acquired."

Not many have published in as many areas as Towns, but he has three masters' degrees in several specializations: Southern Methodist University, M.A. in Educational Philosophy; Dallas Theological Seminary, Th.M. in Systematic Theology; and Garrett Theological Seminary, M.R.E. in Christian Education and Group Dynamics. His doctor's degree is from Fuller Theological Seminary in Evangelism and Church Growth.

Recently, Towns has been writing in the areas of personal renewal and spiritual discipline. He says, "When I first began my ministry in the 1950s, the church needed innovative programs to reach the multitude, so I wrote about church programs. Today our greatest need is spiritual renewal, so I've been writing for personal revival or how to discipline ourselves for spiritual maturity."

Towns wrote *The Names of the Holy Spirit* (Regal Books, 1994), a Gold Medallion winner from the Evangelical Christian Publishers Association and the Christian Booksellers Association. Also under the Regal Books label he has published the fast-selling *Fasting for Spiritual Breakthrough*, *Praying the Lord's Prayer for Spiritual Breakthrough* and *Biblical Meditation for Spiritual Breakthrough*.

11

HEALING CANCER

Interview with

ELMER TOWNS

FAVORITE VERSE ABOUT FASTING:

Is not this the fast that I have chosen? to loose the
bands of wickedness, to undo the heavy burdens, and to
let the oppressed go free, and that ye break every yoke?
Then shall thy light break forth as the morning,
and thine health shall spring forth speedily: and thy
righteousness shall go before thee; the glory of
the Lord shall be thy rereward.
—*Isaiah 58:6,8*

Question: How did you hear about Vernon Brewer's cancer?

Towns: I do not remember who told me that Vernon Brewer
had cancer. I was devastated when I learned Vernon was given
only a short time to live. It was a tragic blow to Vernon, his wife,
Patty, the children and the rest of the Liberty University family.

Question: Why was this such a traumatic event to Liberty students?

Towns: Vernon was the dean of students at Liberty University, and was responsible for the spiritual life of the student body. He administered the discipline when the rules were broken. But in spite of being a person of judgment, the students loved Vernon because he was fair. But more than being fair, they loved him mostly because he was a man of God and he loved them. When the students heard about his cancer, a great sense of gloom set in over the entire campus.

Question: What happened that called all the students to fast?

Towns: Jerry Falwell, chancellor of Liberty University, announced in chapel that we would give ourselves to a day of prayer and fasting for the healing of Vernon Brewer. We designated April 25, 1985, as that day. Dr. Falwell asked that everyone spend at least one hour in intercession for his healing. Falwell reminded us that Jesus had given only one indication how long we should pray. "'Could you not watch with Me one hour?'" (Matt. 26:40, *NKJV*).

Question: How were you involved?

Towns: During chapel of that day, I happened to be sitting next to Vernon Brewer on the platform when the announcement was made that we would be fasting and praying for Vernon's healing. There were approximately 12 leaders from the University sitting on the platform with us: most were vice presidents. President A. P. Guillermin was called to the podium to lead in prayer on behalf of Vernon. As he asked the students to pray, God spoke to my heart—not audibly—God told me to lay hands on Vernon and pray for his healing. My response was:

"No . . . I do not want to do that." I was afraid someone might think I was "Pentecostal." For about five seconds I was worried about what people would say about me. I wouldn't lay hands on Vernon. Then it flashed through my mind,

"Do you want him healed?" God seemed to be saying to me, "Do you really care what people think?"

Instantly, I obeyed God. I placed both hands on Vernon's shoulder, as he was standing to my right. I did not feel anything, as some claim to feel a tingling, or power shooting through their arms and hands when God does a miracle. But in that moment I knew God was going to heal Vernon Brewer.

The Bible describes, "The prayer of faith shall save the sick," (Jas. 5:15). This verse seems to teach us that God gives "the prayer of faith" to certain people to believe Him for healing, and that the "prayer of faith" will heal sickness and turn around a medical condition. As I prayed, I knew God was hearing me, and that He was answering the prayer. By no means do I take credit for Vernon Brewer's healing—5,000 students were praying at the same time. I deeply believe it was the corporate faith of many, not the isolated faith of one person.

Question: Describe the events of the day.

Towns: The food service and cafeteria that feed approximately 3,700 students was shut down on that day. An announcement was made that those who needed to eat because they were diabetic or had some other physical problems would find food on the serving counter. Bread, sandwich spread and drinks were made available. The students were allowed to go into a nearby refrigerator for milk and other foods that were necessary. Because we treat food as medicine for the sick, we expected them to eat.

Question: How many fasted?

Towns: Approximately 3,700 dorm students didn't eat in the University cafeteria that day; only about 50 showed up to eat. The University had approximately 5,500 students at the time. Approximately 1,700 students lived off campus. We did not get an exact number who fasted, but most of the leaders estimated more than 5,000 fasted for that one request on that one day. Most of the faculty and staff joined in fasting, so the number was more than 5,000.

Question: Is there more effectiveness in fasting and praying if a larger number participate?

Towns: God can answer any prayer for just one person; it doesn't take a large number of intercessors to get a prayer answered. But, many strands make a rope much stronger, so having many people pray will strengthen the prayers of one another and stimulate the faith of each other. Jesus said, "Where two or three are gathered...there am I in the midst" (Matt. 18:20), so when many are praying boldly, some of their prayers may not get through because of a personal problem, but others' prayers will be answered.

Question: Describe how the students prayed.

Towns: We asked each student to sign up to pray for one hour at the prayer chapel to intercede for Vernon Brewer's healing. Of course, many students prayed at other places, in addition to praying at the college chapel. The small prayer chapel was open throughout the day. All classes set aside some time to pray for Vernon Brewer. Some classes were canceled for an entire hour of prayer.

I was assigned to lead the prayer in chapel from 2:00 A.M. to 3:00 A.M. It was a warm, lovely spring evening in Lynchburg, Virginia. There was enough of the moonlight when I arrived at the prayer chapel that I saw groups of students clustered in prayer on the lawns surrounding the prayer chapel. Loudspeakers were set up so that what was happening inside was being broadcast outside to the students on the lawn. Even at 2:00 A.M. all the students could not get into the prayer chapel because it seated only 100 worshipers.

A few minutes before 2:00 A.M., I led in prayer, and then read Scripture verses that promised God would hear our prayers if we called unto Him according to His principles. I took less than five minutes to read the verses, sharing the different promises given by God. Then student after student came to the microphone to lead in prayer for those in the chapel, and their prayers were broadcast to those gathered on the lawn.

About half of the students were kneeling at the pews in the prayer chapel, some were sitting, a few were kneeling at the altar. I noticed some of the Korean students were on their faces before God in intense prayer.

I closed in prayer at 3:00 A.M., and the next faculty member took the lead for the next one-hour session. However, when I started across the lawn, one student group after another asked me to pray with them. I did so, praying with the group until all finished praying, and then another group would ask and then another. I did not leave the campus until after 5:00 A.M. that morning.

Question: Did God heal Vernon?

Towns: I wish I could say that God healed Vernon Brewer instantly, but it did not happen that way. First, in an operation the doctors slit open his chest and took out a five-pound cancerous mass. Next, they treated him with radiation, followed by several months of chemotherapy.

Then, to make matters even worse, a terrible accident happened. A needle missed his vein and the medication dripped into his arm and ran down on the inside of his skin into his wrist and hands. It ate the skin off his arm and hand from inside out. Vernon did not need these complications of added fever and terrible side effects. He had to endure skin grafts and several surgeries to repair the hand, all the while battling cancer. So while the healing was not instantaneous—it took over a year—nevertheless, it was miraculous. They predicted he would live for only another three to six months, but, obviously, the prediction was wrong because I see him alive all the time. As a matter of fact, every April 25 I phone him and announce,

"Hello, Vernon . . . isn't it great to be alive?"

God wanted Vernon Brewer to live so he could lead many students into victorious Christian living and demonstrate to them that God can answer their prayers. In 1993, Vernon left Liberty University and founded World Help, a foreign missions organization that plants churches, educates pastors and Christian workers, distributes humanitarian help, and carries out the Great Commission. This multimillion-dollar program takes Liberty

University students and Christians from other colleges on foreign mission trips, getting them involved in missionary work. As a result, many have been called and returned to the mission field. When I look at all of the work Vernon Brewer has done, I understand why God healed him and used the prayer of 5,000 Liberty students to do it.

╡ TAKE-AWAYS ╞

Sometimes the greater the sickness, the greater
the number of people are needed to pray for healing.
Although the prayer of one person can move a mountain
and heal the sick, sometimes there is greater power in
corporate faith and corporate prayer. The faith of many
will encourage one another to more faith and more
prayer, which might lead to greater results.

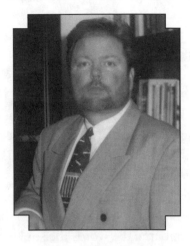

BILL PURVIS

Pastor, Cascade Hills Baptist Church
Columbus, Georgia

The amazing story of the growth and ministry of Cascade Hills Baptist Church, Columbus, Georgia, is reflective of the amazing conversion and ministry of Pastor Bill Purvis. He began pastoring the church on Easter Sunday 1983, when 32 people heard his first sermon. Today, the church averages more than 2,000 each week in attendance. The membership runs at more than 4,000 and the annual income is $2.6 million. The growth has been exponential; they baptized 244 last year and had a total of 520 additions to the church.

When Bill Purvis was an accounting major, a soul winner told him, "Everything you are looking for in life can be found in Jesus." Bill Purvis didn't know how much he would need that statement.

Two weeks later, on April 28, 1974, he picked up a prostitute to try a new experience: after all, he was a young boy from a small Alabama town. It was a setup. The prostitute and pimp were looking for gullible young students to rob. Once inside the room, the pimp took a nine-and-a-half-inch butcher knife and stabbed Bill three times in the chest, neck and liver. The chest wound ruptured his pericardium (sac around the heart), the neck wound cut his jugular vein in half, and according to the doctors he should have died.

Bill ran into the street praying, "Lord, please save me. Forgive my sins. Come into my heart." He thought he was dying and remembered the words the soul winner had told him, "Everything you are looking for can be found in Jesus." While bleeding to death, Purvis prayed and was converted. A friend rushed him to a hospital three blocks away. When Bill walked out of the hospital, he was a new creation in Jesus Christ; his life was radically changed. Since then he has sought the presence of God and built a spiritual church. His influence on the metropolitan area of Columbus, Georgia, gives credibility to his life of prayer and fasting.

Bill indicates that the message to Columbus, Georgia, is the same message the soul winner gave to him before he was saved, and people are responding to that message: "Everything you are looking for in life can be found in Jesus."

﹦ 12 ﹦

A WAY OF LIFE

Interview with

BILL PURVIS

FAVORITE VERSE ABOUT FASTING:

Howbeit this kind goeth not out but by prayer and fasting.
—*Matthew 17:21*

Question: You said, "Fasting has almost been a way of life for me." What do you mean?

Purvis: Several years ago I read the passage that says, "This kind goeth not out but by prayer and fasting." I started thinking about what my prayer life needed. So I added fasting to it. All I knew about fasting was that it began in the evening and went until the next evening. I left off eating a meal for 24 hours and in its place studied the Word of God and prayed. I also heard someone say fasting probably would enhance my knowledge because the blood normally used to go to the stomach to digest food is now being used to go to the brain. So the more I read and prayed during fasting, the more knowledge I felt I could retain.

Question: What specific results have you achieved from prayer and fasting?

Purvis: I started fasting with a friend. His father was a businessman who was not coming to my church. The father had a bad experience with a church deacon and said, "I will never go back." So we started fasting and praying every Tuesday for his father, and as a result his father got saved. About two years ago I looked out into the congregation in our new building, and there was his father. His father attended six months, then told me, "I've come for the last six months and haven't missed a service." He is growing in his faith and on fire for God. God used fasting to show me its power in reclamation.

On another occasion, the church saw God answer prayer and fasting. We were having an outdoor crusade several years ago. We had planned, prayed, prepared and rented an outdoor football stadium. Just when we had everything in place, one of the worst storms to ever hit Georgia was predicted for opening night of the crusade. We had already put 10 or 20 thousand dollars into this crusade. The advertising was out. So I just called our troops to pray, and said, "Tonight through Wednesday we are going to fast all day and pray that God will just turn this storm in a different direction."

Some people said, "Pastor, this is going to be a real miracle." Every time I turned around, I heard more bad news about flooding in areas around us. But we fasted and prayed, and the crusade came. We could see the black sky around the city, but there was nothing but clear weather at the stadium. We went through the entire crusade and God sent great revival. We had a number of folk saved. But the best thing was that people saw the difference fasting made. Some family members drove down from Atlanta, telling us, "We came through the worst storms, we had to pull over to the side of the road because of the heavy rain. We just knew that the crusade was going to be wiped out, but when we got here, there was not a drop of water on us." God used fasting in this case to show the church how to trust Him when things are out of our hands.

Question: When you call the church to fast, what instructions do you give?

Purvis: I ask the people if they are willing to join with me in believing that we need a miracle. I ask them to do without a meal, not to eat breakfast, lunch and supper—three meals. I also ask people to make things right with those toward whom they may have a wrong attitude or to make needed restitution. I tell them fasting isn't going to be some kind of rabbit's foot that makes God give them answers. We don't fast to direct God; we fast to be in a position to be directed by Him.

Question: How did fasting help the church?

Purvis: When the church was small, averaging about 50 people, we didn't have a whole lot of faith. We had no funds. I asked the church to give the largest single offering we could possibly take in one day. The largest offering they could even imagine was about $25,000. So we fasted and prayed for that weekend to produce that amount of money. The offering hit $26,000 that day. God used fasting to show a little church what a big God He is.

Question: Were there other times the church fasted?

Purvis: We fasted about a problem we didn't ask for. When we completed the construction of our new building, the building inspector told us there were some things that we had to tear out and redo. We had to construct different fire walls. They wanted fire dampers behind all the air vents. Even though the inspector had approved the original plans, now he wanted us to tear all these things out and do them differently. Legally, we could have fought him in court, but he wouldn't give us a permit to occupy the building. We were at his mercy.

The total cost of those overruns was $176,000. I told the church rather than fight it in court, and rather than slow down completion, let's just make certain that every contractor doing the work gets paid. For a good name in the community, let's just go ahead and give one single offering to cover the expenses. So we fasted and prayed for that day. The offering was $178,000, two thousand dollars more than we needed. God used fasting to show us that those problems over our heads are still under His feet when we seek Him.

⅀ TAKE-AWAYS ⅀

You can fast and pray about many issues in the life of your church. You can fast for the salvation of the lost, the supply of money, the success of a revival crusade; you can even fast for God to keep a storm away.

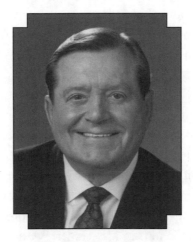

BILL BRIGHT

Founder and President, Campus Crusade International, Inc.
Orlando, Florida

Bill Bright, a former successful businessman, founded and built Campus Crusade International, Inc. into one of the world's largest evangelical organizations, driven by evangelism on the university campus. His influence through Campus Crusade extends into all the world and every part of the Church. While a seminary student at Fuller Theological Seminary in Pasadena, California, the young Bill Bright felt the call of God to share Christ with students on campus at UCLA, an activity that soon became a full-time calling, and which gave birth to the present worldwide ministry of Campus Crusade for Christ.

Of all the anointed tools of Campus Crusade, the *Jesus* film may have presented the message of Christ to more unsaved people than any other form of mass media. As of

April 1998, more than one billion three hundred million people have viewed the film and tens of millions have indicated salvation decisions. It has been translated into more than 440 languages and distributed in 222 countries.

When Bill Bright first wrote and used "The Four Spiritual Laws," he may have given Christians the most-used tool in presenting Christ by personal evangelism ever. More than two billion copies have been distributed in 200-plus languages.

Starting with just Bill and his wife, Vonette, in 1951, the organization he began and still directs now has, in April 1998, more than 16,700 full-time and more than 200,000 trained volunteer staff in 172 countries, and in areas representing 98 percent of the world's population. What began as a campus ministry now covers almost every segment of society, overseeing more than 50 special ministries to inner cities, governments, prisons, families, the military, executives, athletes, women, men and many other segments. Each ministry is designed to help fulfill the Great Commission, Christ's command to carry the gospel around the world (see Matt. 28:19).

⋛ 13 ⋚

CALLING
AMERICA TO
REVIVAL

Interview with

BILL BRIGHT

> FAVORITE VERSE ABOUT FASTING:
>
> This kind can come forth by nothing,
> but by prayer and fasting.
> —*Mark 9:29*

Question: How did God lead you into the ministry of fasting?

Bright: For the past 54 years, I have fasted for different periods of time from one day a week up to four weeks at a time, but I had never fasted for 40 days until God began to work mightily in my spirit in 1993. On July 5, 1994, the Lord called me to begin the first of what has now been five 40-day fasts. After the fast in 1994, God led me to 40-day fasts again in 1995, 1996, 1997 and 1998. These fasts were prompted by the Holy Spirit who was giving me a new and painful awareness of the increasing decadence of our country. For five years God has impressed me to fast and pray for revival in the United States, throughout the world, and for the fulfillment of the Great Commission. I was led to fast and pray because of my urgent sense of desperation for our country. We are losing our national soul. I believe this to be the greatest crisis in the history of our nation. God has impressed me to pray for two million in the United States and Canada who will fast and pray with me for 40 days for national and world revival and the fulfillment of the Great Commission.

Question: What is the most significant answer you have had to prayer and fasting?

Bright: The *Jesus* film was a vision I carried for 33 years before it became a reality in 1979. As of this date, more than one billion three hundred million have viewed the *Jesus* film in more than 440 languages. Tens of millions have received our Lord Jesus Christ.

There have been many significant answers, but standing out in my mind are the great moves of God through the "I Found It" campaign and the gigantic EXPLO gatherings in 1972, 1974 and 1985. Through these events, the Lord mercifully touched tens of millions of lives.

Questions: What has God done for your personal Christian growth through fasting?

Bright: Fasting has drawn me into a more vital, intimate and personal relationship with our Great God, the Father, Son and Holy Spirit through our Lord, Jesus Christ. The Word of God has become even more alive to me. My prayers are more meaningful and effective. Fasting has enabled me to experience an increased joy of the Lord and the power of His resurrection in a new way.

Question: What has God done for your personal worship of Him through fasting?

Bright: These five 40-day fasts beginning in 1994 have brought my worship of God to a new and heightened level never experienced before, even though my walk with God has been very exciting for over 54 years. The times of fasting have greatly sharpened my awareness of His total power and awesomeness, and His great love and mercy.

Question: What experience have you had with others in fasting?

Bright: During and after my first 40-day fast in 1994, the Lord led me to call Christians around the nation to fast and pray. In December 1994, 600 Christian leaders responded to my invitation and met in Orlando, Florida, for three days of fasting and prayer. In 1995, some 3,500 of us gathered in Los Angeles. In 1996 in St. Louis, about 3,700 attended, plus 141 satellite locations joined us from all around the nation. (In 1997, we met in Dallas/Fort Worth with approximately 700 present. However, the major emphasis was on almost 3,000 known TV satellite locations participating.) These were powerful and historic gatherings in the spirit of 2 Chronicles 7:14 as we humbled ourselves, prayed, sought God's face and repented for ourselves and the sins of the nation. There is no doubt that God met with us in a special way.

Question: What are the typical experiences you follow when fasting?

Bright: First, I set a specific objective. If the Lord leads us to fast, He will usually burden our hearts with an objective. We should prayerfully ascertain what that is so that our efforts may be focused. My major focus is for national and world revival and the fulfillment of the Great Commission.

Second, I prepare myself spiritually to seek God's face, not His hand. The very foundation of fasting and prayer is repentance. Unconfessed sin hinders our prayers. In Scripture, God always requires His people to repent of their sins before He will hear their prayers. So with God's help I search my heart to make sure there is no unconfessed sin in my life.

The third step is to prepare myself physically. We should not rush into a fast. It is helpful to begin by eating smaller meals before we abstain all together. This sends our minds a signal that we have entered the time of the fast, and it helps to "shrink" our stomachs and appetites. I must confess, however, that I have not always followed this practice personally.

Some health professionals suggest eating only raw foods for two days before starting a fast. Preparing ourselves physically makes the drastic change in our eating routine a little easier; then we can turn our full attention to the Lord in prayer.

Fourth, I ask the Holy Spirit to enable me to experience a meaningful fast as I seek God's face. He honors a humble and contrite spirit.

Question: What direction would you give to a person who has never fasted?

Bright: Our fasts should always include plenty of water or they can be life threatening. People with certain physical and medical problems should never fast without professional super-vision. If there is any doubt, a physician should always be con-sulted.

If a person has never fasted, I recommend he or she start with shorter fasts of one meal a day, or one day a week, or one week a month to develop "fasting muscles" before attempting a 40-day fast. Anyone who fasts and prays should seek to restrict regular activity during the fast in order to truly seek God's face. The person should also be prepared for the spiritual "battle." Prayer with fasting is not always easy and in some measure involves spiritual warfare, but there is no victory without a bat-tle. Our eyes should be kept on Jesus, and the victory will sure-ly come. Remember Satan has no power over us apart from what God allows.

Question: How would you prepare a group of people for fasting?

Bright: Each person should be advised of the above principles, and more, as contained in one of my books about fasting, such as *The Coming Revival.* Group fasting should have a common purpose, and the leader should instruct all the group members about adequate cautions, preparations and suggestions, and help maintain focus during the time of fasting and prayer.

≩ TAKE-AWAYS ≨

> You should follow proven guidelines when fasting; this way you join the tradition of others who have successfully fasted. You should be sincere, be committed, be prepared and be faithful to God. When you fast in faith, God will direct your prayers and reward you (see Phil. 2:13).

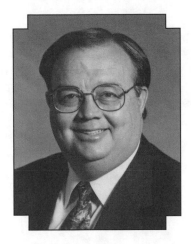

RON PHILLIPS

Pastor, Central Baptist Church
Hixson (Greater Chattanooga), Tennessee

Ron Phillips has pastored Central Baptist Church for 20 years, where a tremendous increase in attendance of more than 2,000 a week has occurred. Under his leadership, the church has added millions of dollars in buildings. But the greatest growth is in spiritual renewal and evangelism. God's power is upon Phillips when he preaches. In the year they began fasting, 535 members were added; that doesn't include many others who came to Christ and joined other churches.

Phillips has held most state and national offices in the Southern Baptist Convention and graduated from Southern Baptist Convention higher educational institutions, earning his doctor's degree from New Orleans Baptist Theological Seminary. Phillips preaches weekly on "The

Central Message," the televised ministry of his church's Sunday messages, which are shown on a national and international network. He has published nine books with Evangel Press, Pathway Press and other publishers.

14

FASTING FOR REVIVAL AND RENEWAL

Interview with
RON PHILLIPS

FAVORITE VERSE ABOUT FASTING:

If my people, which are called by my name, shall humble themselves, and pray, and seek my face, and turn from their wicked ways; then will I hear from heaven, and will forgive their sin, and will heal their land.

—*2 Chronicles 7:14*

Question: How did you get into the ministry of fasting?

Phillips: After a one-day seminar by Elmer Towns in my church about "Fasting for Spiritual Breakthrough," 123 members of Central Baptist Church committed themselves to fast for at least one day a month for revival and soul-winning outreach. At the conclusion of the seminar, I organized those who made a commitment to fast, so that each day of each month was covered by one person fasting and praying, and some days there were as many as six people fasting (most people committed themselves to fast once a week). They fasted and prayed for soul-winning outreach until the annual Christmas drama called *The Book* was performed, written by Fred Guilbert, our minister of music. Then revival broke out.

Originally, our church planned a six-night choir and drama presentation for our Christmas pageant. But so many people were saved that the program was extended for a total of 14 performances. One hundred fifty-three people were converted in just one service alone, and a total of 998 prayed to receive Christ.

Question: What other results did the church experience because of fasting and prayer?

Phillips: Sunday School attendance jumped to 287 people, church attendance jumped to more than 410 people, offerings jumped $550,000 for the month of December over the same month in the previous year, and the church had an all-time record of baptisms.

The church had held its previous fall revival in October before we began fasting, resulting in only 28 professions of faith, but God opened up heaven and poured out His power through our Christmas program. The church spent $28,000 for the program for laser lights, costuming, advertising and a full dramatic presentation.

Those who attended the Christmas musical/drama at Central Baptist Church of Hixson were expecting Christmas carols, three wise men, a star and baby Jesus. What they got was a heart-pounding, eye-opening, destiny-altering look at the Holy One, the evil one and the reality of heaven and hell.

The Christmas program was scheduled for six performances, tickets were printed for crowd control, and an extensive advertising campaign was planned. However, before the printed and television advertising could hit the marketplace, all but a few hundred tickets were gone. Word had already spread that this program was going to be different.

Thirty minutes before the ninth performance, and what was supposed to be the final performance, was to begin, the auditorium had to be closed. Two hundred people were placed in a makeshift overflow area and hundreds of people were turned away.

After an orchestral overture, the lights came up on the auditorium. The actors entered from the back of the sanctuary in character and costumes as late arrivals to the performance. They sat as spectators during Act I. In Act II they went onto the stage, and that set the stage for Act III. During Act III, the actors were called to appear to meet God before a gigantic throne. As they walked forward, the voice of Satan could be heard over the sound system, "This one is mine . . . ." After the *Book of Life* was opened, they heard the voice of God pronounce, "Depart from me ye cursed . . . I never knew you." And then they were thrown into a gaping hole in front of the audience; fire, smoke and screams gushed out of hell.

We gave the invitation in an unusual way. We had the people bow their heads in prayer and receive Christ as Savior. I told them, "If you meant business, then please stand up." Then, with every new Christian standing, I asked them to follow the pastoral staff out the side door, where they were told how to begin the Christian life. Each evening as the unsaved people departed, there was thunderous applause from the audience showing approval of the decisions made for Christ. One area church baptized 21 new people into its membership, just because its members had brought unsaved people to see our Christmas program.

Question: What is your church's next fast challenge?

Phillips: I am going to challenge our church to a Daniel Fast beginning Sunday, August 17. I am challenging the church to fast for several crucial issues. Scripturally, the Daniel Fast was over a long period of time. He had received the prophecy of God's long-range plan for Israel. We as a church need to fast to find out what God's long-range plan is for the continuation and growth of our ministry. We'll begin with the Lord's Table on Sunday evening and that will launch the fast. Some will be fasting 7 days, some 14 days, some will do the total Daniel Fast 21 days, and a few people may feel led to do the full 40-day fast. We believe God will bring us as a church into our destiny and out of our wilderness in many areas of our ministries. This is the third fast we've called since we began our first one when Elmer Towns challenged our church to fast.

Question: What will be involved in this fast?

Phillips: Basically, we're asking our members to eliminate all pleasure party foods; that includes breads, cakes, etc. Some will be led to use unleavened bread (cracker type bread). But no leavened bread, no cakes, cookies . . . all meat will be eliminated . . . and we're eliminating of course any alcoholic beverages. We're asking people to stay strictly with healthy foods because the Daniel Fast is a fast for health. Many have weight situations that can be helped with this fast. Not only are we fasting to get the vision, but also to be healthy. We're asking people to limit themselves to vegetables, juices . . . if they have to eat, we're suggesting vegetables, to eat them raw, or some people will boil cabbage and that kind of thing. It's really a little more strict than a total Daniel Fast in that we're asking people to use a little soup, juice or mixed raw vegetables.

Question: What are you going to do in the way of corporate prayer meetings?

Phillips: We have a number of small groups that are going to organize themselves in prayer. We will be having a special season of prayer at the end of 7, 14 and 21 days, and of course at the end of the fortieth day. Basically, we're going to wrap up this campaign the third Sunday in September. I'll still be in the fast but most of the people will be off by then. We will have a victory Sunday. At the same time we have been working all summer with architects, with leadership services and with other leadership advisors to develop our plans. We hope to come to agreement on a master plan. We're fasting to have God's Word on this. Hopefully, early in October the vision will be crystal clear to all.

We'll be presenting to the congregation our plans for church growth, prayer plans and mission plans for the next 10 years.

Question: What are the physical things for which you are fasting?

Phillips: Our challenge to fast involves paying off the indebtedness of another 12 acres of land the church just bought. We now have 30 acres that connect us with the mall parking lot. That gives us a direct road into the mall parking lot, which extends our future indefinitely at this site. We're going to be looking at a new worship center, not because we couldn't expand with multiservices, but we believe we have to become a state-of-the-art arena where drama, video, music and TV ministry can be combined in a larger setting that can minister to our entire city. We had about 40,000 people visit the church in three weeks, so we believe that our ministry needs a larger auditorium. We need a 3,700-seat arena that can be expanded to 5,000 persons for special events, but we also need to close it down to 2,500 seating for smaller events.

Question: What typical experiences do you follow when you're fasting?

Phillips: The first three days and sometimes the fourth day I find myself obsessed by thoughts of food. I find my best comfort is taking prayer walks. I do not just sit around; I go walking in the neighborhood to pray. After the third or fourth day, the physical struggle ends.

Then I am able to focus on my study of the Word and I find new truths as I read the Scriptures. I begin to get words from God and I am able to hear God out of Scriptures in a clearer fashion. The Scriptures come more alive. Putting together a sermon and writing it usually takes six hours, but I can accomplish it in an hour and a half or two hours while fasting. When I am fasting, time speeds up and I can do more things more quickly that relate to ministry. When working on sermons, Bible study or a book, these projects come together more quickly when I am fasting.

On the ninth or tenth day, I have euphoria, almost a druglike state—perhaps it's because the last of the poisons are leaving the system. I drink distilled water during the fast. I stay away from tap water with chlorine because when I'm fasting my body is more sensitive to any kind of drug or chemical. I drink fresh fruit juices, fresh vegetable juices and plenty of water. I also have an energy rush. This is kind of dangerous because I think I can go and play 18 holes of golf, but I can't. If I go the full 40 days, my physical activities will be limited.

I find myself emotional when fasting. The least thoughts about Jesus bring tears or laughter to me. I find spiritual things seem more precious, like hearing hymns—every word rings in my spirit and brings tears of joy to my eyes. I feel a closer relationship or intimacy to Jesus.

Question: How do you break a fast?

Phillips: I start eating soft foods, primarily vegetable soup with a little meat stock. I tell my church members not to go out and wolf down a cheeseburger. It will make them sick. Basically, it is best to add food slowly to the diet. I learned my lesson that if I try to eat a heavy meal within four or five days of ending a fast, I'll make myself sick.

≩ TAKE-AWAYS ≩

You can bring revival to your church by praying and fasting. The more people who fast and pray, the greater the revival, and the longer they fast and pray, the greater the revival. Ron Phillips's church experienced a great demonstration of power in soul winning because the core workers fasted for revival and prayed for an evangelistic outreach. However, a leader has to cast the vision of revival and a leader has to organize the people to pray, as was the case with Ron Phillips.

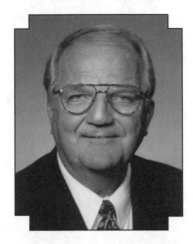

LEROY L. LEBECK
Senior Pastor, Assemblies of God
Trinity Life Center
Sacramento, California

Leroy Lebeck has pastored Trinity Life Center for six years. Trinity Life Center has a congregation of more than 1,700, and the congregation meets in the facilities built on 17 acres. The dream of a new sanctuary was fulfilled when in November 1997 the congregation moved into the new 2,400-seat sanctuary. Trinity Life Center houses a Christian day school that includes grades K–8. Lebeck is also president of Trinity Life Bible College, founded in 1972.

Lebeck graduated from Bethany Bible College, Santa Cruz, California, in 1957 with a B.A. degree. He became the pastor of the Pentecostal Tabernacle in Kitamat, British Columbia, Canada, from 1959 to 1961. There he met Marilyn Miller, who would become his wife. In 1962 they were elected to serve as pastors of the Richmond Pentecostal Tabernacle in Richmond, British Columbia. In December 1966 they accepted a missionary appointment with Overseas Missions Department of the Pentecostal Assemblies of Canada, and served in the West Indies. They taught in the West Indies School of Theology in Trinidad. In 1972 they returned to Canada to pastor the Christian Life Assembly in Langley, British Columbia. During his 10-year tenure, the church grew from 120 to 1,800 in attendance. Pastor Lebeck conducted weekly television programs on the British Columbia Television Network.

15

A NEW SPIRITUAL ENERGY LEVEL

Interview with

LEROY L. LEBECK

FAVORITE VERSE ABOUT FASTING:

Is not this the fast that I have chosen?...and thine health
shall spring forth speedily.
—*Isaiah 58:6,8*

Question: What do you enjoy about fasting?

Lebeck: One of the things I enjoy the most about fasting is that I really rest during the fast. I renew my strength and renew my spirit. I don't go to work; that means I don't go into the church. I stay at home and finally get rest. I don't eat and I get tired when I fast. I yield to that and go to sleep. When I get up, I read my Bible and read Christian books. When I get weary again, I let myself go to sleep. I have a hot tub out in the backyard. I sit in the Jacuzzi and read, pray, relax outside in a chair, and enjoy the sunshine. The days I spend fasting, there is a tremendous recouping of my strength and physical energy. It really seems to be a Sabbath. It is a kind of fast—A Sabbath Fast.

Question: Besides the fellowship, what else does God do for you?

Lebeck: Every time I fast, I renew my spiritual energy level that comes when I feel He is anointing me. When I speak, I need an unction from the Lord. When God anoints me, I am more communicative with people. After that when I walk down the street, people seem to smile at me. I can return the smile and feel a positive blessing that God has smiled upon my life. I feel blessed and that I can be a blessing.

Question: How did God lead you into the ministry of fasting?

Lebeck: I really didn't do a lot of fasting until I read a book by Lee Bueno called *Fast: Easier Way to Health.* It is taken from Isaiah 58:8, "And thine health shall spring forth speedily." Bueno quotes nature itself, showing that animals fast when they are sick. They don't go to the hospital; they just fast to get better. They just quit eating when they are sick. So we humans can learn something from them.

Question: So you look forward to fasting?

Lebeck: There are many reasons to fast. I have led the church to fast for healing, for miracles and for the power of God. There have been times when we fast because of spiritual warfare. These are times of intense intercession.

Question: But fasting also has an enjoyable side.

Lebeck: Yes, fasting is a time to read and restore my spirit; a time to meditate and clear my mind; a time to be physically refreshed because I rest and sleep; a time to cleanse my body so I'll be renewed for the work of God.

Question: What are the benefits of fasting?

Lebeck: When Jesus talked about fasting, He said in Matthew 6:4, "Your Father who sees in secret will Himself reward you openly" *(NKJV).* Some of the benefits I have found in fasting are found in Isaiah 58. Some of those rewards Isaiah promised have come to my life through fasting and prayer. In verse 6 it speaks of being set free from "the bands of wickedness." Burdens are lifted, the oppressed go free and yokes are broken. "Then your light shall break forth like the morning, your healing shall spring forth speedily" (v. 8, *NKJV*). The *NIV* version reads, "your healing will quickly appear."

I have just come off a 40-day fast and I have never felt better. This was a juice fast and I can truly say I never battled hunger, but felt healthier every day. I juiced vegetables so that there was no loss of enzymes and vitamins, and also juiced fresh fruit. One of the benefits was a much-needed weight loss of 25 pounds.

Another benefit I find through fasting is answer to prayer. Isaiah 58:9 says, "Then you shall call, and the Lord will answer; you shall cry, and He will say, 'Here I am'" *(NKJV)*.

I highly recommend fasting and prayer. It is not always convenient, but the rewards are worth it.

≩ TAKE-AWAYS ≩

You don't need to fear fasting. There are some enjoyable sides of fasting if you will look for them and plan for them. You can be physically renewed by fasting, as well as spiritually renewed. In life you usually get what you seek, so seek a well-rounded healthy life—emotionally, mentally, physically and, of course, spiritually.

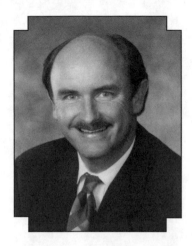

DANIEL HENDERSON
Pastor, Arcade Baptist Church
Sacramento, California

Daniel Henderson is the senior pastor of the 2,000-member Arcade Baptist Church, which is known for its spiritual commitment more than its physical assets ($2.8 million annual budget). Henderson is a recognized leader in prayer among the pastors of Sacramento and provides prayer/leadership with his association of Conservative Baptist churches at a regional and national level.

Daniel was student body president at Liberty University before joining the staff to become pastoral training coordinator. He left Liberty University with a team of 13 to plant Cornerstone Community Baptist Church in Greater Seattle and built the church to more than 400 in weekly attendance.

Henderson became executive director to the Masters Fellowship for John MacArthur in Newhall, California, but the attraction of the pastorate was too great. He feels God has called him to a ministry of spiritual renewal through prayer summits, renewal and fasting. He received the honorary doctor of divinity degree from Liberty University in 1990.

16

TEACHING FASTING TO A CHURCH

Interview with

DANIEL HENDERSON

FAVORITE VERSE ABOUT FASTING:

Is not this the fast that I have chosen? to loose the bands
of wickedness, to undo the heavy burdens, and to let the
oppressed go free, and that ye break every yoke?
—*Isaiah 58:6*

Question: Tell me about the first time you entered into a fast.
Henderson: I fasted several times for a day or two when I was in
seminary. The most memorable fast happened when I was preparing
to move to the Northwest to plant a church. I was scheduled to begin
the church the following spring and the new college year was just
starting. I was still single. I really did not have peace about going into
some new dating relationship just to get married because I was start-

ing a church. I was really torn. I prayed, "Lord, do you want me to go start this church as a single man?" I began to fast just to get peace from God and a sense of direction. I began a 21-day fast. Through some events that were really beyond my control, and the persuasion of a friend, I agreed to go on one date with this girl. Before the 21-day fast was over, she and I felt that God wanted us to get married. Funny as it sounds, through this 21-day fast, I found my wife.

Question: Tell us what you did on those days of fasting.

Henderson: One of the difficulties was that I was in school, yet fasting doesn't require total shutdown of a schedule. I set aside every mealtime to be alone with the Lord. I spent some extra time early in the morning and, of course, most evenings in prayer and reflection. I restricted my diet to clear liquids such as diluted apple juice, diluted broth, water . . . those kinds of things. I tried to maximize every available moment that would have otherwise been spent eating meals, just to be with the Lord.

Question: How did you fast as you began the church?

Henderson: Before we planted the church, I again did a 21-day fast. I spent time just asking God for His wisdom and His empowerment. We were getting ready to move with a team of 14 adults and several children to the Northwest. We had two semi-trucks full of furniture. Starting from scratch, not knowing anyone, we felt this was certainly something far beyond what we could accomplish on our own. This was really a fast for the empowerment and provision of God.

Question: I had heard that Yonggi Cho, the pastor of the world's largest church in Seoul, Korea, had challenged Liberty students who were going to start a church to spend 10 days fasting before beginning a church. Did you accept this challenge?

Henderson: Yes, in fact, the challenge of Cho triggered me not only to fast before we started our church, but also to fast about the whole issue of going as a single man versus waiting. Should I wait until I was married? It was a very difficult issue that only God could solve.

Question: What happens to you when you fast?

Henderson: I have found that fasting recalibrates vision, appetite, desire and focus. I can really trace back my own hunger for the Lord and my desire for prayer as being regularly linked to the times of fasting in which I set aside those moments to be with Him. Fasting is a time to focus my appetite on Him. Hunger for God really challenges us spiritually, more than any physical thing.

Fasting enhances the joy of time spent in His presence. It causes all the passages of Scripture that speak of hungering after God and thirsting after Him to come alive. Two fasts while I was in school were done with others. The first fast I did was with Rick Amato. Rick was a very tense, fiery student evangelist. He and I actually fasted during those 21 days and spent time in prayer together. The second fast was conducted in conjunction with the team that was going with me to start the church.

Question: What did you gain by fasting with others?

Henderson: Accountability and encouragement are two of the great assets of fasting with someone. You join in spirit and desire for God and you share prayer answers together in what the Lord is teaching.

This Sunday my congregation is sponsoring a churchwide day of prayer and fasting. We are launching a $5-million-dollar capital campaign in our church. We will have a daylong emphasis on prayer and fasting. Throughout the morning, there will be prayer meetings going on as they always are during the services. As soon as the worship service is over, we will go right into the service of worship and prayer together that will conclude with the communion service.

Question: How do you prepare a congregation for fasting?

Henderson: Obviously, I have taught fasting from the pulpit. I think it is important they understand the biblical foundation of fasting. We also encourage them to do some reading. We have pamphlets available. We also have books in our church library. We remind them of the heart behind fasting. In fact, this coming

Sunday as part of my message I am referencing Isaiah 58, which talks about the fast. It is not just a matter of going through a religious ritual, but really having our hearts changed and having our compassion for people deepened and being broken before the Lord. I review with them the heart attitude behind fasting so it doesn't become a religious ritual.

Question: Does having a corporate goal in front of the people play a role in getting people to fast together?

Henderson: Every fast ought to have some goal. Sometimes only the Lord knows the goal when He puts certain things inside our hearts. But in most fasts, God reveals a goal clearly to us. In our particular case, the goal is to have our faith strengthened and for our hearts to be open with a vision for what God can do in our church in the next eight weeks. In particular, we need to yield to the Lord, including our financial resources. We are fasting to see God do a good work in our hearts. We need a new spirit of generosity and commitment to the vision that is put before us.

≹ TAKE-AWAYS ≸

You need to let God touch you through fasting before you can lead a church or group to fast. Fasting will give your group unity of spirit before God gives financial or material results. Usually, the secret of a fasting church is a leader who fasts and prays.

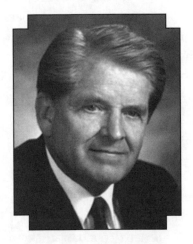

WILLIAM T. GREIG

Chairman and Publisher
Gospel Light Publications/Regal Books
Ventura, California

William T. Greig is chairman and publisher of Gospel Light Publications. He is a visionary with a heart for the evangelization of the world. Well known in the Christian community as a world Christian and champion of excellence in Christian education, Bill Greig has been actively involved in Christian publishing for more than 50 years.

He began his career in Minneapolis, Minnesota, in 1946, following his separation from the U.S. Navy. Prior to joining the Gospel Light team as vice president in 1950, Bill Greig was partner/manager of Praise Book Publications in Minnesota. In 1972, he was elected president of Gospel Light by the board of directors.

Bill Greig has served in key leadership roles for organ-

izations vital to the ministry of Sunday School and
Christian education. He has previously been president of
the National Sunday School Association, and was a founding director and past president of the Evangelical Christian
Publishers Association. He was also a founder and president of the Minnesota Sunday School Association, and has
been actively involved in the Sunday School movement as
a Sunday School superintendent and teacher since the
early 1940s.

Mr. Greig presently serves several agencies as a trustee:
GLINT (Gospel Literature International); St. Petersburg
(Russia) Christian Publishing; Concerts of Prayer Inter-
national; John M. Perkins Foundation; Joy of Living Bible
Studies; and the International Reconciliation Coalition.

Married for 47 years, Bill and his wife, Doris, who is the
founder (and author of many of the studies) of the Joy of
Living Bible Studies program, make their home in Ventura,
California. They have four children: Kathy, who is director
of Joy of Living; Bill III, who is president and CEO of
Gospel Light; Gary, who is associate professor of Hebrew
and Old Testament at Regent University's School of
Divinity in Virginia Beach, Virginia; and Jane, who is the
producer of Gospel Light Video. The Greigs continue to be
actively involved in the Community Presbyterian Church
where Bill serves as an elder, and he is active with the Love
Ventura County pastors' prayer fellowship.

17

GAINING
SPIRITUAL
INSIGHT

Interview with
WILLIAM T. GREIG

> ### FAVORITE VERSE ABOUT FASTING:
> "If my people, who are called by my name, will humble themselves and pray and seek my face and turn from their wicked ways, then will I hear from heaven and will forgive their sin and will heal their land."
> —*2 Chronicles 7:14, NIV*

Question: What motivated you to undertake a 40-day fast?

Greig: I had become too much of a professional Christian. I did things that I was supposed to do. I attended meetings I needed to attend, and went about my Christian activities doing appropriate things. I think I may have lost my first love. But while on my first 40-day fast, I became more sensitive to other people, both Christians and non-Christians, and especially to God who prompted me with Isaiah 30:21 *(NIV)*: "Whether you turn to the right or to the left, your ears will hear a voice behind you, saying, 'This is the way; walk in it.'" As I became hungry, or craved something good to eat, God prompted me to pray for people, some of whom I had never met (i.e., while I was driving, I would see teens walking along the street, other drivers, families, etc.). As I prayed for revival in my own life, my church, my city and my neighbors, I became more open and available to God's Holy Spirit and more sensitive to what He wanted. I began to hear His promptings and experienced some divine appointments with people He wanted me to talk with.

Question: What events led up to your 40-day fast?

Greig: My wife and I had been in Orlando, Florida, and had dinner one evening with our longtime friend Bill Bright of Campus Crusade for Christ. I had heard Bill advocate fasting, and now he shared with us his experiences of three 40-day fasts. On his first, he had fasted to lose weight, and for spiritual reasons. He said the Lord had shown him it was not a valid reason to fast. Meantime, all I could think to myself was: *Maybe he did it, but I could never do even one day, let alone 40!*

On the jet headed back to California, I read a book by Bill Bright in which he called on Christians to fast for spiritual breakthrough and revival. I had heard how Jerry Falwell did a 40-day fast, drinking water and taking Centrum vitamin pills daily. And how, after 25 days, he did another 40-day fast for the financial survival of Liberty University without telling anyone else the reason for his second fast. While I marveled at it, I was sure it was impossible for me. But then God spoke to me in that "still, small voice" and said, "Just do it! Try it. I'll help you."

I resolved to obey, and started the fast before we touched down at Los Angeles International Airport. Immediately, I gained strength from the decision. I have never looked back to wonder if I made the right decision, though I often wondered,

Can I hold out? Whenever I had that question, I would pray and thank the Lord that I could in His strength. As I report this, I am in the thirty-seventh day of my second 40-day fast in response to Bill Bright's request for two million Christians to join him in praying for revival and the evangelization of the lost. (It's going great, too!)

Before my second 40-day fast, at my wife's insistence, I talked with our family doctor. Earlier the previous year I had foot surgery and carelessly got an infection that put me into the hospital for a second surgery—my first hospital stay in my 73 years. The Lord brought me through what could have been a serious problem. God has answered my family's and my prayers for both physical healing and spiritual strength. I believe they would agree that God has answered their prayers on my behalf both physically and spiritually.

Question: What was your daily intake?

Greig: In addition to taking vitamins and minerals, as suggested by our doctor, each morning I drink Slim Fast blended with fresh fruit and ice cubes, often with some low-fat milk. When I go out to lunch I often drink tomato or V-8 juice, iced tea (with lemon) or coffee, and occasionally hot or cold broth or soup. The same is true for supper. When friends note my liquid diet, they often look puzzled. I am reluctant to tell them I am fasting lest they take it as spiritual pride, which in turn makes them feel guilty. Usually they comment: "I could never fast!" or "My health wouldn't allow it!" or "I've always wanted to lose weight, but simply can't fast." I often quote Bill Bright that losing weight is not a worthy reason for a spiritual fast.

When people seem uneasy that I am not eating with them, I assure them I am not really hungry, and that their eating doesn't bother me at all! (Though I occasionally admit I am often tempted by the steak, pancakes, toast, pie, cake, or you name it.) The fact is that for me fasting is not so much what I eat (or drink), but what I don't eat—that which I deny myself! That is the spiritual discipline where the blessing starts. And when I crave something that way, I pray for whatever God lays on my heart at that moment. I pray for repentance, revival and new commitment in the Church in order that we may experience a sweeping revival in our city, state, nation and around the world, especially the 10/40 Window.

Question: What did you learn during the fast?

Greig: I have begun to learn self-denial. I thoroughly enjoy eating; and no wonder, my wife, Doris, was a home-economics teacher and is a fabulous cook. Over the years I added 35 pounds, which I didn't need. Those pounds made it harder to ride my bike up hills (we live on the hillside) and my inherited knee problems were aggravated, making stairs a problem. Now, on the thirty-seventh day (of my second 40-day fast), and almost our forty-seventh wedding anniversary, I am back to the weight when I was married in 1951. I really didn't try to lose weight, though it is a little serendipity from the Lord who knew I would feel better and continue to be more active without the extra weight. I learned a new meaning from Luke 12:22 and 23.

Best of all, I am beginning to learn to "pray without ceasing," in season and out of season. I am seeing needs in people I was previously unaware of: neighbors, friends, rebel kids, pious and "holier than thou" types, etc. I was previously indifferent to, or worse, almost contemptuous, of street people, druggies, gays, or hard but broken people, etc. The Lord is beginning to let me see them through His eyes, and feel their pain as He does. Or I'd see a church, New Agers or a cultic center, with which I wholly disagreed on a biblical basis, and I would think a judgment on them. Not so now; He moves me to pray for their release from Satan's deception and bondage, and their coming to Christ.

Before fasting, I would prayerwalk our neighborhood each morning praying for families, neighbors who drove by, and people in general. Now I am meeting and getting to know individuals and their needs, the illnesses in their families, the broken relationships, the New-Age group that meets across the street each week, the father who is not a believer who told me "he's different!" when I asked about his son who has a Jesus sign on his car. The son had been delivered from a severe drug addiction in a group led by my nephew. His father was not pleased that he had become a believer, so now I can pray intelligently for the son and his parents who obviously don't know the Lord.

I had prayed generally for a retired couple who live across the street from our church parking lot. They have never visited the church, as far as I know. One day before 7:00 A.M. as I walked by, I heard, "How are you doing?" It was from a man, about my age, having his first cigarette of the day on the front porch. I went over and introduced myself and said a few words. As I left I said, "Have a good day and God bless you!" Subsequently, I stop to chat, and he is very friendly. He is retired form the U.S. Navy, where I served in World War II. We hit it off. He introduced me to his wife and we have a friendly relationship. I keep praying specifically for an opportunity to share Christ with them and invite them to our home for fellowship. It was one of those divine appointments that the man started by greeting me. Now we have a good friendship and I pray that God will lead me to the next step for both him and his wife.

Question: What else did you pray for during your 40-day fast?

Greig: When I get to the top of the hill at the end of our street, there is a panoramic view of our entire city, which lies along the shore of the Pacific Ocean. I can see the Channel Islands, which reflect on the beauty of God's marvelous creation . . . the green mountains, blue ocean, white breakers, lovely islands, flowers, birds, trees, etc. It is truly breathtaking! But now I do more than thank God for His wondrous creation! I am aware of how easy it is to become "at ease in Zion" and forget the tragic plight of so many children, youth, families and individuals living in this beautiful place. The children are too often neglected or abused, the youth into drugs or demonic activities, the single parents are struggling, and most have no hope and much pain with little, if any, knowledge of Christ.

I see many good churches, yet so removed from life as it is really lived down there, and many believing Christians virtually lulled to complacency by the beauty of God's creation, caring little about the plight of their neighbors. This moves me to pray for revival to come to our church, to every church, and to see the evangelization of our city, county, state and nation. Ventura, California, is a lovely place, but so many of our neighbors are no less lost than the people in inner-city America.

Question: What has the 40-day fast done for Gospel Light?

Greig: It had never occurred to me to fast and pray for our sales, but I am frequently reminded to pray for the countless thousands of pastors, churches, Sunday Schools, teachers, families, children and youth who use our products every week.

I pray for a new vision from God for our management team and for our product design and development people who create the products we sell. I pray for vision, spiritual sensitivity, a commitment to prayer as a regular part of our process, and sincerely seek God's guidance for everything we do. When I realize the number of Sunday Schools and vacation Bible schools we serve, we pray for their revival and for the millions of children, youth, adults and families they reach. We pray that every vacation Bible school and Sunday School will be an avenue of outreach to unchurched families in their neighborhood. It is sobering and makes us realize our utter dependence upon God so we can truly make a difference here in America and all around the world where our Regal and Renew books, curriculum and other resources are translated and published in more than 100 languages. This can be accomplished only by prayer and total reliance upon God.

Our mission at Gospel Light came to us from Henrietta Mears, our founder. It was over the teaching lectern at the Hollywood Presbyterian Church for the 36 years she taught the college department class. It was there as a reminder for every member, as well as the teacher: To know Christ and make Him known!

＝ TAKE-AWAYS ＝

You will get spiritual insight by fasting and praying. You will see people through the eyes of God and you will see their spiritual needs. While you may be afraid to begin a 40-day fast, you will get strength from that decision, and God will help you complete the fast for the glory of God.

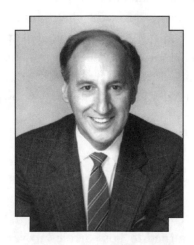

JACK HAYFORD
Senior Pastor, The Church On The Way
Van Nuys, California

Jack W. Hayford is the senior pastor of The Church On The Way, Van Nuys, California. What began as a temporary assignment to pastor 18 people in 1969 has continued fruitfully, and today the congregation numbers more than 9,000 members, and has an amalgamate weekly attendance approaching 10,000.

Hayford has become a recognized statesman for God, being called upon by many services for opinion, insight and counsel. His insight into God's Word and an uncompromising commitment to practical application characterize Pastor Hayford's teaching. During his long tenure as a senior pastor of one local church, he has become recognized for his balance in preaching, and avoiding extremes, while not diluting or compromising truth. Hayford graciously reveals the heart of a holy and merciful God in all his sermons. His deep commitment to spirituality gives him a unique credibility to discuss fasting in this volume. His travels and ministry to denominational and interdenominational gatherings at colleges, seminaries and parachurch organizations have caused Pastor Hayford to become an acknowledged bridge builder—helping forge healthy bonds among all sectors of the Church.

Jack met Anna Smith in college and they were married in 1954. After they both graduated with honors from LIFE Bible College in Los Angeles, California, they began their ministry in Fort Wayne, Indiana (1956-1960). From that pastorate, they returned to Los Angeles to serve as national youth directors for the International Church of the Foursquare Gospel (1960-1965). During the next eight years, Jack served on the faculty of LIFE (1965-1973). Later, from 1977 to 1982, he served as president of LIFE Bible College, while simultaneously serving in his pastorate at The Church On The Way.

The Church On The Way is one of the leading megachurches of America featuring multiple services. In 1987, the church bought the facilities of the First Baptist Church of Van Nuys, four blocks away. The congregation was able to double by using both auditoriums for simultaneous Sunday morning worship services. Hayford preaches in both services.

⇥ 18 ⇤

FASTING
IS SPIRITUAL
WARFARE

Interview with

JACK HAYFORD

> FAVORITE VERSE ABOUT FASTING:
> "This kind does not go out except by prayer and fasting."
> —*Matthew 17:21, NKJV*

Question: What motivated you to think about fasting?

Hayford: I began to awaken to the power of fasting through two passages of Scripture. The first is in Daniel where he saw the promise of Jeremiah (see Dan. 9:10,11) that the people would be delivered after 70 years of captivity and returned to the Promised Land. The text reveals how Daniel recognized that God's promise was true, but that it needed to be appropriated with prayer. In essence, Daniel said in chapter 10, "Thy word was true, but the warfare against the evil one was strong." Daniel began a fast, but as he fasted evidence came that an obstacle was keeping him from realizing the fulfillment of God's promise. The obstacle was a blockage in the spiritual realm caused by demonic beings opposed to the purpose of God. What was intended by God to be "loosed" on earth was being "bound" in the invisible realm—against God's will and promise. But the power of demons was broken through Daniel's fasting and prayer. This is consistent with Jesus' teaching. He enunciates this principle about spiritual warfare in the New Testament, showing how fasting may "release" God's will by breaking through demonic obstacles: "This kind does not go out except by prayer and fasting" (Matt. 17:21; see also Mark 9:28).

Here the disciples, in essence, ask Jesus, "Why can't we cast out the demon from the boy?" (Mark 9:28). Jesus' answer: "Pray and fast!" So these two passages—an Old Testament text and a New Testament one—give strong evidence that fasting holds great potential as an instrument of spiritual warfare.

Question: Why is fasting an instrument in spiritual warfare?

Hayford: I don't think anyone can explain how fasting works in this warfare, but that it works is clear in the Word—and Jesus' words on the subject are "why" enough for me. He says, "This kind of demon is evicted by this means." How? I don't know. But there is something about fasting that apparently drains the capacity of the adversary to resist. So that's basically why I think we should employ fasting with prayer—for example, in concern for our nation.

Question: How does your congregation fast?

Hayford: In November 1973, the Lord dealt with us very strongly on an unforgettably profound Wednesday night service. We sensed Him calling us as a congregation to pray for our nation as a long-term assignment, and continue to fast and pray most Wednesdays—to this day. At that time, we took the promise of 2 Chronicles 7:14: "If My people who are called by My name will humble themselves, and pray and seek My face, and turn from their wicked ways, then I will hear from heaven, and will forgive their sin and heal their land" *(NKJV).* We started convening our Wednesday night service at 7:14 P.M. instead of 7:30 P.M. (note the time is 7:14 P.M. not 7:15). This helped us focus internally on the promise of God's Word, and our call—to intercede—for our nation. Later, as we got into regular intercession, we found it began to take more time, so now we start the service at 7:00 P.M., though we will sustain the "7:14" concept. But intercession for the nation was really how we got started in fasting.

Question: What are other ways your church fasts?

Hayford: We almost every year observe one or two "believer's fasts." This is a three-day fast where the congregation is encouraged to fast with a specific focus, and many of the congregation do it. For example, we often observe the three-day fast on the Sunday through Wednesday preceding Thanksgiving Day. We'll start on Sunday night, observing the Lord's Table together. We'll worship the Lord, and set our focus for prayer. Because it is all in the spirit of thanksgiving, we launch with prayer at the Lord's Table. Then we encourage believers to let the next meal they eat be Wednesday night in the evening. Some people, of course, will observe it with a partial fast, but together we agree to pray for special evangelistic or other spiritual points of breakthrough—family issues, job circumstances, etc. We also apply Isaiah 58:6,7, and aim for a great Thanksgiving offering, converting the money we saved on food while fasting to a gift of love to feed the hungry—both spiritually and physically needy.

(Note: By breaking the fast on Wednesday evening, we urge people to begin reestablishing their body's normal digestive operations before they have a Thanksgiving meal. We've never had any physical repercussions from people who suffered from this fast, and we have had great, great spiritual breakthroughs!)

We will often lead our people to fast in days preceding Good Friday. I have often personally observed a three-day fast from Wednesday to Friday leading up to Good Friday. It sobers my own soul for the coming celebration of the Cross, and I believe it holds enriching potential for believers.

Finally, as a general practice, and on a regular and continuing basis in our congregation, Wednesday is considered to be a day of fasting. People observe it to different degrees, but many of our people fast on three days of the week, then gather for power-prayer at the evening service.

≣ TAKE-AWAYS ≩

You can fast to prepare yourself for the true meaning of Thanksgiving and the Easter season. You can also fast regularly to know God and walk with Him. When you fast, you may protect yourself or others from the evil one because fasting and prayer can break his wicked hold over you and your desires, or the bondage that holds others captive.

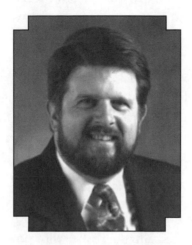

GARY GREIG

Associate Professor of Hebrew and Old Testament
Regent University's School of Divinity
Virginia Beach, Virginia

Gary Greig is a favorite professor at Regent University and also serves as senior consulting editor for Gospel Light/Regal Books. As a son of William T. Greig Jr., chairman and publisher of Gospel Light/Regal Books, he also has a rich heritage in Christian publications that extends back to his great-aunt, Henrietta Mears, founder of Gospel Light. Greig graduated from the Hebrew University of Jerusalem, where he received his master's and doctorate in Near Eastern Languages and Civilizations. Greig is fluent in modern Hebrew and proficient in German, French and Spanish.

Greig wants to help believers understand the biblical and theological basis of the present ministry of the Holy Spirit with healing, miraculous spiritual gifts and "signs and wonders." He is cofounder of Love Ventura County, a fellowship of 80 pastors who pray and work together to reach the county for Christ.

Gary Greig wrote the Regal release *The Kingdom and the Power*, a collection of 13 essays based on solid exegetical studies by well-known and respected evangelical theologians and church leaders. It was a joint editorial effort with Kevin Springer, pastor of Vineyard Christian Fellowship in Palm Desert, California. *The Kingdom and the Power* provides Christians from every denominational background an opportunity to examine the charismatic gifts for themselves. Compelling evidence is presented that God desires His Church to proclaim the gospel with power and to minister with all spiritual gifts . . . today.

OVERCOMING FEAR BY FASTING

Interview with

GARY GREIG

FAVORITE VERSE ABOUT FASTING:

"Is this not the fast that I have chosen: to loose the bonds of wickedness, to undo the heavy burdens, to let the oppressed go free, and that you break every yoke? Is it not to share your bread with the hungry, and that you bring to your house the poor who are cast out; when you see the naked, that you cover him, and not hide yourself from your own flesh? Then your light shall break forth like the morning, your healing shall spring forth speedily, and your righteousness shall go before you; the glory of the Lord shall be your rear guard."

—Isaiah 58:6-8, NKJV

Question: Tell me about the first time you fasted.

Greig: That was about five or six years ago. I don't remember all of the details exactly but it was for a day. I read about fasting in Peter Wagner's books and began to fast once a week. At first it was pretty tough because I got dizzy and tired. But the sense of God's presence was wonderful. Then I couldn't wait every week just to get close to the Lord. I fasted to grow in the Lord and to seek and receive more anointing for what God would have me do. I was fasting for other people, healing, deliverance and various situations for which I was praying.

Question: What type of opposition have you had in fasting?

Greig: Before I moved to Virginia, a couple of instances come to mind. I remember the Lord said to me, "I want you to fast this day about a house in Virginia. I'll provide a house for you if you will just seek My face." I didn't want any difficulties in all of the possible business complications that come with buying a house, so for two or three weeks I spent the whole day fasting and praying, asking God to provide us a home and to let the transition be smooth. And our move was the smoothest transition. We could have ended up staying in an apartment for months until we got into a house, but it wasn't that way. When we moved, the time frame fit us. I am convinced that because I obeyed the Lord and sought Him in prayer and fasting, the transition was smooth. I believe spiritual warfare would have opposed us and made it difficult to get into the right house.

Question: Do you have any barriers to fasting more than one day?

Greig: I don't have much trouble being tempted by food when I am fasting. What is hard for me is to get started and I'm tempted at the end when I know I'm coming out of a fast. During the fast, I shut down my desire for food and it's not as hard for me to go without food. My biggest challenge is to get over the threshold of starting a fast. If I can get myself through the first couple of hours that I am going to fast, I am fine. I obeyed the prompting of the Lord to do a 21-day fast last spring. The hardest part was getting into the fast. I had fears. I had questions. "Am I going to make it?" I even feel that way about a one-day fast. I always question if I am going to make it. Will I have enough strength? Maybe I have fears because I always end up getting a little dizzy or out of balance physically.

Question: What is the greatest thing you've gotten from fasting?

Greig: I am used to being a second son in the middle of the family. For various reasons, I think it makes me a fearful person. On my 21-day fast, the Lord took me back and showed me our Jewish grandfather from Czechoslovakia. He and his family converted to Christianity and became a part of a reformed church in Czechoslovakia. He went through much persecution, which we know from family records. My fears were nothing compared to what he must have felt. God had said to start praying about my fear. The Lord had me lift my fears up to Him in prayer. It is hard to describe, but I felt a peace coming on me in the twenty-first day of my fast. From that time to this, I have never struggled with that latent fear I used to have about every circumstance. That fear was always hanging around every situation I was in. I would always become afraid of worst-case scenarios. It was just an atmosphere of fear. It left me . . . I am free of that. I know the difference between what I used to feel and how I feel now. I feel free.

⅔ TAKE-AWAYS ⅔

You can have your greatest emotional fears taken away by prayer and fasting. But remember, the greater the fear, the more you will have to fast and pray, and the longer you will have to fast and pray. God can deliver you from all your fears.

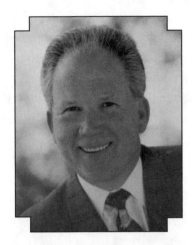

DALE E. GALLOWAY

Dean, Beeson International Center
for Biblical Preaching and Church Leadership
Asbury Theological Seminary
Wilmore, Kentucky

Dale Galloway became dean of Asbury Theological Seminary's Beeson International Center for Biblical Preaching and Church Leadership in 1995, leaving the pastorate of New Hope Community Church, Portland, Oregon, a church he founded. Galloway was an innovative pacesetter in small-group ministry in Portland, following the example of Yonggi Cho, who planted the largest church in the world by using small, home-cell groups. Galloway taught a seminar across the United States about small-cell ministry. When he saw the potential of this seminar to train church leaders, he began considering a move to Asbury Seminary.

Galloway is the author of more than a dozen books including *20-20 Vision* and *The Small Group Book*. During his 23 years at New Hope, the church grew to 6,400 members, 80 percent of whom were previously unchurched. The church's need-meeting, pastoral-care-providing small groups averaged 5,500 in total weekly attendance. Galloway trained more than 500 lay leaders to lead the small groups of his church.

He received his academic training from Olivet University, Kankakee, Illinois, and Nazarene Theological Seminary, Kansas City, Missouri, and was honored with a doctorate from Western Evangelical Seminary, Portland, Oregon.

FASTING ABOUT A DIFFICULT DECISION

Interview with
DALE GALLOWAY

FAVORITE VERSE ABOUT FASTING:

"Ask, and it will be given to you; seek, and you will find;
knock, and it will be opened to you."
—*Matthew 7:7, NKJV*

Question: Tell me about your first experience with fasting.

Galloway: My first experience with fasting was when I saw my mother fasting. She would fast and pray because she was very concerned about my older brother who was five years older than I. She was fasting very intensely for his salvation. I saw her heart break over the actions and life of my brother. That was one

of the things God used to bring me to Himself. My older brother hasn't come to Christ yet. God used my mother's fasting and
prayers to bring me to Himself and into ministry.

Question: Tell me about one of the first occasions you
remember fasting.

Galloway: As a pastor in my first church, I began fasting and
praying that God would teach me to be a soul winner. I was
going door-to-door planting a church, and I didn't know how to
win souls. So I began to fast and pray about the matter. I read a
book by Gene Edward, *How to Have a Soul-winning Church*,
and continued fasting and praying about how to lead someone
to Christ. God brought Gordon Walker into my life at Olivet
University. As we sat in the student union, he showed me in a
few minutes how to use "The Four Spiritual Laws" to lead a person to Christ. That very afternoon I led two people to Christ. I
had been calling in homes without results, but with that simple
plan, I applied "The Four Spiritual Laws" and they worked. In the
next few weeks, I led more than 35 people to Christ using that
plan. This was about 35 years ago. I was planting the Grove City
(Ohio) Nazarene Church, which has become a great church in
that denomination under some outstanding pastors. But the
church's foundation was built on prayer and fasting.

Question: What other significant answers to prayer have you
had when fasting?

Galloway: When I was starting New Hope Community
Church, Portland, Oregon, in 1972, we had no money and no
people. It was a very frightening time in my life. My wife and I
fasted and prayed for God to give us that city and to help us
learn how to reach unchurched people for Christ.

Question: You planted and built New Life Community
Church into a congregation of more than 5,000 people. Was it
difficult to leave the position of pastoring people you loved and
led to Christ, and move to Kentucky to assume a position in aca-
demics, becoming the dean of the Beeson International Center

for Biblical Preaching and Church Leadership at Asbury Theological Seminary?

Galloway: When I face difficult decisions, like coming to Asbury, I pray and fast. I pray for God's will to be done in my life. By fasting, it becomes important to break or humble ourselves before God, so we're not looking for our own advantage or advancement. By fasting, I was seeking God's will more than wanting my own will. I came to a place where I was crying out to God for help in this decision. It was a very emotional experience. I was so attached and committed to building the church in Portland that I had a hard time letting go. It wasn't an instant decision, but a long-term process as I continued to fast and pray. The decision took about a year to make. It required time for me to be willing to let go of that ministry and open myself up to a new ministry.

Even at the time I doubted whether I was doing the right thing. But on the other hand, God had spoken to me and God had led me in response to fasting and prayer. Until I came to Asbury and saw what assets I had, and what opportunities I had, I realized then I did the right thing.

Now I can extend my pastorate through many young people who are trained at Asbury. I can love my students as I loved my people back in Portland, Oregon, and they love me and my family. Instead of pastoring just one church, I am influencing hundreds of churches. Perhaps one day I could influence thousands of churches by influencing those who will pastor churches. All of my life has been in preparation for this ministry. As I look back, I can see it was a long process that God used to bring me to Asbury. It was a long process of prayer, fasting and seeking His will.

TAKE-AWAYS

You can solve two issues that face you by prayer
and fasting. First, you can become a soul winner by
asking God to teach you how to do it and asking God to
help you lead people to Christ. Second, you can make
difficult decisions by constant fasting and prayer.
Sometimes the answer does not come instantly,
nor does the early morning sun rise instantly.
But when we have difficult decisions to make,
the answer usually comes slowly like the first rays
of the sun, and gradually we see God's answer as we
wait before Him in prayer and fasting.

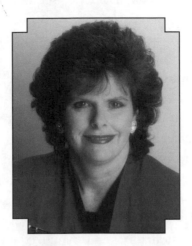

CINDY JACOBS
President and Cofounder
Generals of Intercession
Colorado Springs, Colorado

Cindy Jacobs has often been called a "spiritual warfare specialist." She travels in many nations meeting with leaders and intercessors to confront spiritual strongholds over their cities, states and nations.

Cindy is president and cofounder of Generals of Intercession, a missionary organization devoted to training in the area of prayer and spiritual warfare. The Generals of Intercession staff believes that prayer truly changes things, and that without it this world will not be won for the Lord. The ministry is currently involved with the United Prayer Track of A.D. 2000, under the leadership of C. Peter Wagner, to see that every unreached people group of the world (about 6,000 people groups in all) are receiving strategic prayer by the year 2000 in order to see them reached with the gospel.

In September 1985, the Lord spoke to Cindy and her husband, Mike, to gather the "generals of intercession" to pray for the United States. After several meetings throughout the United States, the Lord expanded this vision to other nations. As these generals have gathered throughout the world (England, France, Argentina, Israel and Russia), the Lord has revealed His battle plans in prayer through each one bringing a part of the strategy.

Cindy is also the international advisor-at-large for Women's Aglow Fellowship and serves as a member of Aglow's International Prayer Council. She has currently taken on the coordinating/leadership position for the U.S. Spiritual Warfare Network. This network of ministry leaders strategize for the United States on the spiritual warfare prayer level, seeking national revival. She also serves as a director for March for Jesus.

Cindy Jacobs's second book, entitled *The Voice of God*, was published by Regal Books. She recently authored her third book, *Women of Destiny*, also with Regal Books. Her first book, *Possessing the Gates of the Enemy: A Training Manual for Militant Intercession*, was published by Chosen Books.

21

FIVE SPECIFIC REQUESTS

Interview with

CINDY JACOBS

FAVORITE VERSE ABOUT FASTING:

Sanctify ye a fast, call a solemn assembly, gather the
elders and all the inhabitants of the land into the house
of the Lord your God, and cry unto the Lord.
—*Joel 1:14*

Question: What is the greatest thing you have seen from fasting?

Jacobs: This year I went on a long fast and it ended as I ministered in a church in Louisville, Kentucky. In that meeting, there were many miracles that came as a result of fasting, both my fasting and a corporate fast by the church. One woman said that two chambers of her heart didn't beat together, but she was totally healed during that meeting. Many people were dramatically born again, family members were restored to fellowship.

Question: What type of fast was it?

Jacobs: It was a corporate fast where the whole church prayed for five specific things . . . for 25 percent increase in financial income per year, for healing, for household salvation, for freedom from addictions and for permanent weight loss. I have found that anything that affects the whole church catches my heart. The whole church fasted and prayed for these five things and the whole church experienced the work of God.

Question: Did the whole church fast with you?

Jacobs: Yes, the whole church was called to a fast . . . they do this every year . . . some members fast for 21 days. The church has been fasting every January for eight years in a row. They keep pictures on big boards of lost loved ones for whom they are praying. They organize so that someone is praying each hour of every day while they're fasting. I believe they're praying in a prayer room at church. One lady's daughter-in-law who was an exotic stripper was dramatically born again while I was speaking at the church. The people had prayed years for her.

They also fasted and prayed that people would lose weight and keep it off. They were able to maintain their weight loss by a program of fasting.

Question: How do you get ready for a fast?

Jacobs: I usually start preparing by eating less. Then I begin to prepare myself spiritually. I begin to ask God for verses to claim as promises for answers to prayer. Then I begin to prepare myself mentally for what's ahead. Recently, we needed a major financial breakthrough for our ministry. On the twentieth day of fasting, we had the largest contribution we had ever received. We received this incredible breakthrough in answer to prayer and fasting. A man I had not previously met phoned one day and asked to have dinner with my husband and me. He gave our ministry the largest donation we have ever received.

Question: When you're in a fast, what do you take?

Jacobs: Sometimes I take vitamins; this fast I just took juice (fruit and vegetable). Because I was traveling a lot during that time, I had to adjust to the things I can do. First of all I pray and ask God what kind of fast would please Him. And then I do that kind of fast.

Question: What kind of fast do you follow?

Jacobs: There are several kinds of fasts: the Daniel Fast (only vegetables); a total fast (without any food, only water); the Esther Fast (without water for a couple of days) is a spiritual warfare fast. For me the type of fast depends upon the severity of the situation. When I fast for dedication I ask the Lord what He wants me to do. Sometimes in my heart I don't feel love for God as much as I used to. If I feel my heart is growing cold, I will go on a more severe fast. To really hear and seek God, for my own intimacy, I will fast longer or I will withhold more.

Question: Describe what you mean by the Esther Fast against spiritual warfare.

Jacobs: Well, I find out that all hell breaks out before all heaven breaks loose. When I begin to fast, Satan does everything emotionally to stop the fast. Like me, you'll find things won't work in your family, you'll sometimes feel a little bit depressed, not always from the physical side, but because Satan is fighting you. He doesn't want you to believe in God for answers to prayer. If Satan can get you to feel terrible you easily believe that fasting doesn't work. So you have to press through that first cycle of attack. Usually for me it's the first week. After that I can intercede. And in the last week Satan will attack again. The last week is very difficult for me.

Question: How do you break a fast?

Jacobs: Well, it depends upon the kind of fast. I take consommé, something very light, no salad, no potato. Actually, there are very good recipes that will help get your digestion going again. You can actually harm yourself by breaking a fast the wrong way. I have a friend in Indiana who fasted for 40 days, then ate Chinese food to end the fast. He was hospitalized that night.

Question: How would you instruct someone to begin fasting?

Jacobs: I would tell them to begin gradually. First, lay off caffeine. Learn to get through that, then abstain from other food. Find a prayer partner to pray with you. Please the Lord from the heart. I would try a day or three days at the beginning. The key is pleasing God's heart; fasting is not a work of the flesh.

Question: What are some other practices you follow with fasting?

Jacobs: I fast at least one day every week. Also, I have a covenantal fast going with other families. We pray for them every Wednesday morning as we fast that day. In return, they are fasting and praying for our family. Our fast is our gift to each other.

Question: What other insights do you have about fasting?

Jacobs: I think our flesh is a very poor conduit for the Spirit of God to use in speaking to us, although God does speak to us through our bodies. But remember, the flesh is not a friend of the Spirit. Fasting really can purify us and get us ready to hear the voice of God; just as some things are good conductors of light, fasting is a good conduit for godliness. God speaks to us when we fast.

₃ TAKE-AWAYS ₎

You can fast with others to get greater
results from God. You can fast with a church
congregation, or you can have a covenantal fast with
another family. When you fast, ask God to give you a
goal; you might have several goals for which to fast.
Cindy Jacobs fasted for five specific requests.

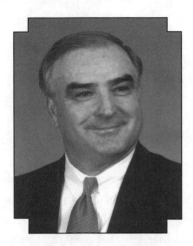

TOM MULLINS
Pastor, Christ Fellowship
Palm Beach Gardens, Florida

Tom Mullins pastors Christ Fellowship, a church he planted in 1983, which has grown to 3,200-plus (weekend) and
4,000 (weekly) attendance. The church has $2 million in
facilities, and has just purchased 20 acres at $2 million
(other 20 acres in option) for expansion. An 1,800-seat
sanctuary is being built for $8 million. All this happened
in 15 years. The church converted a horse barn and riding
arena into one of the most beautiful sanctuaries, which
ministers to the elite who live nearby, yet draws all sections of society from a large metropolitan area.

Tom Mullins was not trained as a minister, but rather
spent 15 years as a football coach. His teams averaged nine
victories a season and earned number-one ranking in the
high schools of Florida. He went on to coach in college.

Watching Tom Mullins in ministry is not seeing your typical minister in action. To him, pastoring is coaching people to love Jesus and to get excited to live for Him. His preaching is like a half-time locker room exhortation—full of passion and enthusiasm. His pastoral counseling is like coaching a player on the sidelines preparing to enter the game. He trains his pastoral staff and lay leaders as he would a football huddle preparing for the next play.

The spiritual passion and zeal of Tom Mullins, and his people, have been the driving forces that built this church—more than methods, programs and techniques. Because Tom has committed himself to know God and His power, he is qualified to have his testimony included in this book.

22

RESPONDING TO THE CALL OF FULL-TIME SERVICE

Interview with

TOM MULLINS

FAVORITE VERSE ABOUT FASTING:

If my people, which are called by my name, shall humble
themselves, and pray, and seek my face, and turn from
their wicked ways; then will I hear from heaven, and will
forgive their sin, and will heal their land.
—*2 Chronicles 7:14*

Question: Tell me about how you began fasting.

Mullins: I entered into this discipline of fasting about 13 or 14 years ago. It was at a pivotal point in my life. I was trying to decide whether or not I was going to go into the business world or stay in athletics where I had great success. Also, I was wrestling with the call to full-time ministry. Now I believe God really called me into ministry as a teenager, through my grandfather's ministry. I believe my grandfather's mantle was passed to me. But for years that mantle lay on the shelf and I didn't pick it up. However, from the time I left for college, I have been ministering somewhere in a church every weekend. I was either leading singing, working with young people or speaking. For years, I served in the state of Kentucky as an interim pastor for many churches that were between pastors.

December 1983 was the crisis point in my life. I was in Israel when I felt God was issuing that call again. I felt in my spirit that if I did not respond to God's call, I might not receive that call again. That's when I yielded everything. I said, "Lord, whatever you want me to do . . . even if being a pastor . . . I will do it." To be honest, I did not want to be a pastor. It was a frightening sense of responsibility and accountability. I had an awesome fear of God, but I didn't want to grieve Him.

Question: What grew out of this experience?

Mullins: Fasting grew out of this experience. I came to the realization that some things only come through prayer and fasting. I remembered that my grandfather taught and preached fasting. But fasting was never a major part of my life until I answered the call.

As a little boy I remember asking my grandfather why he wasn't eating. He would say that he was fasting. Fasting was something that was never taught much, but my grandfather fasted when he was seeking the face of God. When I fast, I get all the static out of my thinking and I get rid of all the other mixed signals in my life. I get to the purity of God's voice and listen to His "still small voice."

I fast because I have a hunger to be absolutely in the center of God's will. When God brought me to a breaking point where I surrendered my own desires, that's when I began fasting.

Question: Who was your grandfather?

Mullins: He was Tom Steenbergen, a minister of the gospel in the Church of God, Anderson, Indiana (Wesleyan Holiness). His primary focus was on pastoral ministry. He was a pioneer in many areas. He helped establish many major camp meetings in Pennsylvania, Kentucky and Ohio. In his early years, he traveled as an evangelist; his song evangelist was Dale Oldham, father of the well-known gospel singer Doug Oldham who is carrying on the ministry of his father today. Dale was a major influence in our family. My middle name is Dale, named after Dale Oldham. Tom is my first name, named after my grandfather.

Question: What was the first fast connected with the growth of this church?

Mullins: My first fast was really whether or not I would birth this church. I fasted to know if it was God's will. So my wife and I declared a time of fasting and prayer to get spiritual insight into God's will. Out of the blue I got two or three phone calls from established churches that wanted me to come be their pastor. I had not received calls like that for many years. When I got those calls, they all came around the same time . . . within a few days of each other. At that time I said to my wife, Donna, "This is highly unusual. Could God be in this?" We continued praying and fasting. At the same time, people were telling us that God wanted us to birth a church. All these pressures drove me to fasting.

Question: What has been your continued practice of fasting?

Mullins: I began fasting one day a week early in the ministry of this church. Then I got excited about it and started fasting two days, Saturday and Sunday. But I had trouble fasting on those days, then trying to preach on Sunday. I found that following a two-day fast, it was physically and emotionally difficult. So I backed off from fasting every weekend and found myself fasting for special occasions and special prayer requests.

Question: What has been the most outstanding result of fasting?

Mullins: I think the building we have today comes from prayer and fasting. Our church is a horse barn that has been converted into a worship center through the work of the people. The ministry has literally exploded in the last four years as a result of fasting and prayer. We also bathed this project in prayer and fasting as we built it. This was the result of an old-fashioned kind of barn-raising effort by all the people. I was construction coordinator, but the church had men that would meet with me every morning around 6:00 A.M. before they would go to work. We would pray right on these grounds, six days a week, for God to bring in the laborers that day.

Question: What did God do for this church?

Mullins: This sanctuary is worth $2 million, but we paid only $400,000. This horse barn was a preexisting steel structure with a roof. It was 20 years old and the building department certified it was sound, so we were able to build up and around it. The people basically did so much labor on this project that its cost was minimal.

As we prayed, miraculously God sent in men with labor skills, and materials that amounted to hundreds of thousand of dollars of savings for us. As soon as the barn got finished, God started bringing in the sheaves. Church attendance doubled the day we opened the doors; the next year attendance doubled again. The following year we doubled again. The fourth year we doubled again and now attendance is running between 3,200 plus people that worship with us in five weekend services (two on Saturday and three on Sunday morning).

Question: How is your daily schedule altered when you fast?

Mullins: Normally, I don't alter my daily schedule much, except for the fast. I usually eliminate solid foods for that fast day. Then I try to take the time I normally spend at lunch to focus on prayer. For me, I have to get away from the office to pray. The office is the hardest place in the world to pray because of the interruptions. I have to walk and pray. Every time I have a desire for food, or to satisfy my physical needs, I try to reflect in prayer.

Question: How do you prepare your people to fast?

Mullins: One time I asked our people to fast TV for a week. I asked them to spend that time with their family. Make it a time when they studied the Word of God with their families. We had tremendous results from that week. The only bad thing about that week . . . it was the biggest football game in the state—Florida was playing Florida State, and they went on to become national champions. Remember, I used to be a football coach, so that made it difficult. I didn't know the game was on that weekend and I longed to see it, but I did not neglect that fast.

≩ TAKE-AWAYS ≨

When facing a major decision—Tom Mullins faced a major decision about his vocational future—you may need to fast and pray for God to show you His plan for your life. When you truly fast, you stop feeding your physical and material nature and let God feed your soul. Then, in your emptiness, God can tell you what He wants you to know. God can show you what He wants you to do, and God can reveal what He wants you to become.

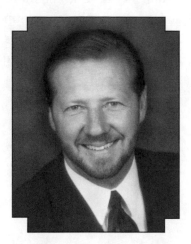

DUTCH SHEETS

Senior Pastor
Springs Harvest Fellowship
Colorado Springs, Colorado

Dutch Sheets is the senior pastor of Springs Harvest Fellowship in Colorado Springs, Colorado. He has dedicated his life to training others for ministry, has served on the faculty of Christ for the Nations Institute, and is currently an instructor for Christian Life School of Theology, Colorado. He serves as an advisor on the National Board of Aglow International and is also a guest lecturer at Fuller Theological Seminary. He has traveled extensively ministering to the Body of Christ throughout the United States, Canada, Central America, Africa and much of Europe.

His congregation calls him Pastor Dutch. His book *Intercessory Prayer*, as well as several audiotape series, has extended his ministry beyond the limitations of physical presence and/or travel. His commitment to fasting supports his total ministry objectives. His newest book with Regal Books is titled *The River of God*.

23

FASTING WITH YOUR CHURCH FOR GOALS

Interview with
DUTCH SHEETS

> ### FAVORITE VERSE ABOUT FASTING:
>
> Then shall thy light break forth as the morning,
> and thine health shall spring forth speedily: and thy
> righteousness shall go before thee; the glory of the
> Lord shall be thy rereward.
> —*Isaiah 58:8*

Question: What is the greatest thing God has ever done for you through fasting?

Sheets: The greatest thing God did for me was on a 21-day fast. At the end of the fast, God opened to me a great revelation I had never seen before. It was a new dimension of understanding of God and His word, a new understanding of how God wanted me to walk. I am teaching things today as a result of the fast. Whenever I share these things with people, they are touched and God ministers to them through that truth.

Question: How do you prepare for a fast?

Sheets: I try to enter the season by withdrawing from activities, not just food, but activities and mental stress, so I am not dealing with these issues on the first part of my fast. You know, a fast is difficult enough physically that I don't want to have to deal with these issues as I start withdrawing, and preparing myself physically and emotionally. I slow down and get into the mood, and prepare my frame of mind to make me more conducive to what God wants to do.

Question: Do you write down what you learn in a journal?

Sheets: I've never been good at that. I always have goals in my heart when I fast. On one occasion I did not follow that; I didn't know why the Lord wanted me to fast. It was only that God so strongly impressed me to fast. But typically, I believe that one should have specific goals and it's always good to write them down.

Question: Tell me how you prepare a group for a fast.

Sheets: I begin with a season of teaching, a lengthy season. A few weeks ago I prepared my people by asking them to prepare their hearts for what they're going to do for God this year. I gave them a few instructions to physically get them ready to fast, and I tried to encourage them to begin making preparation for fasting.

Question: When you fast, what are your personal habits about drinking and nourishment?

Sheets: Physically, the first thing I try to do is get longer periods of rest. I decrease my activities as much as possible. When I have a busy ministry schedule or obligations with my family, I don't try to fast during these obligations. I try to do what everyone teaches: drink lot of liquids. When I fast solid foods, I drink juices, and lots of water. I just try to pour the liquids in.

Question: Do you drink coffee?

Sheets: No coffee on the fast. I used to drink caffeinated coffee; now I drink only decaffeinated. But when I did drink it, during the first few days of my fast, I had to wean myself from caffeine. The first days of the fast I might have a couple cups of coffee to keep headaches from happening. Now I just drink juices, or if I'm fasting all foods including fruit juices, I just drink water.

Question: What day of the week do you fast?

Sheets: I try to fast regularly, but I do not pick the same day of the week. I'll fast sometimes for a day, sometimes for two to three days; often I'll just fast a meal. But I do not have a regular, systematic day to fast.

Question: What do you say to people in your church who have physical problems such as diabetes?

Sheets: I tell them they must absolutely get counsel and permission from their physicians. Do not try to fast totally without the advice and counsel of a physician. I try to release them from any condemnation or guilt they may have because others are fasting and they feel they must do it. Sometimes a doctor will tell people they can't do it. I support the doctor's opinion. But there are many kinds of biblical fasts and there is something each person can do. Maybe they can do a Daniel Fast where they eat only certain foods. I remind them that God will honor that. If their physician is not given to spiritual things or doesn't understand this, I encourage them to find one, even if it's not their regular physician.

Question: When the church was fasting together, did you try to begin and end together?

Sheets: We began the fast together; the church started on a weekend. I shared with them the things that we were going to be asking from the Lord. We did not end our fast with any kind of a celebration. But I think we should have. Looking back on it, that's a great idea. In fact, I would try to give them some instructions in writing the next time we fast. I will try to give them something to encourage them and share excitement, just because they came through the fast. Next time I probably would have a celebration service at the end.

Question: Your church just finished a 21-day fast. What was the purpose of the fast?

Sheets: We set five goals. Here is the list I shared with my people:

1. We fasted for spiritual cleansing in our midst—personal holiness.
2. We prayed for revival in the church.
3. We asked for a demonstration of God's miraculous love.
4. We fasted and prayed for souls to be saved, i.e., the harvest.
5. We asked God to provide land. We're seeking the Lord to show us where we should relocate.

≡ TAKE-AWAYS ≡

Some people approach fasting systematically by
writing their goals, keeping a journal and joining
with others to begin and end together. Other people
let the Lord lead them in praying and fellowshipping
with Himself. Both approaches are blessed by God.
Although Dutch Sheets was sensitive to God's leading,
he also had five major requests for which he led
his church to fast and pray.

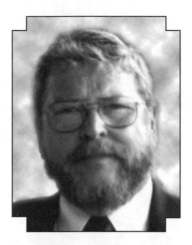

DONALD RAY STUKEY

Layman
St. Peter's Lutheran Church
Fort Pierce, Florida

Donald Ray Stukey is a layman who lives in Fort Pierce, Florida. He is an eight-year member of St. Peter's Lutheran Church and was formerly a United Methodist. He firmly believes in the power of prayer and fasting and has witnessed what he considers to be miracles and healings.

24

SOLVING CHURCH FINANCIAL PROBLEMS BY FASTING

Interview with

DONALD RAY STUKEY

FAVORITE VERSE ABOUT FASTING:

And I set my face unto the Lord God, to seek by prayer and supplications, with fasting, and sackcloth, and ashes.
—*Daniel 9:3*

Question: How did St. Peter's Lutheran Church begin fasting?

Stukey: Our experience with prayer and fasting started about six years ago. The pastor, Rev. Ted Rice, preached messages for four weeks on stewardship. At the end of the fourth message, he asked people to try tithing for three months. His part of the bargain was to stay in the sanctuary for the next three days in prayer and fasting for each of those who agreed to tithe. Then he prayed for them each morning for the next 87 days. The church income went from $104,000 a year to about $220,000.

Unfortunately, the church had some severe problems that went back many years and pastors. Things got bad enough that Pastor Rice felt a great need to go to God for serious help. So he did a 40-day fast to call on the Lord. God responded by removing negative people from the congregation. To make a long story short, "We are now a wonderful, loving church that is seeking God's will for our lives and our church."

Question: How did the property sell in response to fasting and prayer?

Stukey: Because a number of people left, two years ago during the month of July, we were short of funds. At the council meeting that month, someone said we needed to cut out some things because we could not pay all our bills. Pastor Rice said we were not going to cut anything. What the church would do was to have a 24-hour prayer and fasting session. The pastor and the church council met in the sanctuary on Friday at 6:00 P.M. until Saturday at 6:00 P.M. We planned to seek the Lord as a church.

We reminded God that we tithe to our synod and because of His promises in Malachi 3. We had the best income in July we had ever had, enough to carry us through the summer months with no problem. The following week a major drugstore chain offered us $1.3 million dollars for our property. We settled for $1.4 million. This was a real blessing because we had only 3.5 acres and an old building that needed a lot of help. Now the church owns 18.6 acres almost next to the exit to the interstate and the church is planning an 18,000-square-foot building. God is faithful and able to do what He says.

Question: Were there other illustrations of fasting?

Stukey: The story continues. Everyone in the city of Fort

Pierce told us that the sale would never go through, that our old property would never be zoned commercial by the zoning board or the city commission. The members of my church suggested prayer and fasting. God gave us a great victory.

We continue to fast for other victories and God is faithful.

⩺ TAKE-AWAYS ⩻

A church can fast for tangible items such as finances and the sale of its property. Even when God began to answer prayer, the people needed to continue fasting because there were other obstacles to selling their property.

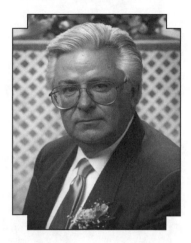

LESTER F. AYARS
Senior Pastor, Northport Baptist Church
East Northport (Long Island), New York

Lester Ayars has been senior pastor of the approximately 1,000 people of Northport Baptist Church for 30 years. The church has grown significantly under his ministry, more than in members, budget and resources; its significant growth has been in its spiritual effect on the members. Although the church has grown in physical properties to several millions of dollars, its greater assets are the young people sent into ministry, and families that have been grounded in the faith who have been transferred from this Greater New York City location.

Ayars is a graduate of Moody Bible Institute, and has transitioned the church from traditional worship and Sunday School to become a predominant cell church having a strong praise worship format.

25

LEADING
THE CHURCH
TO FAST

Interview with
LES AYARS

FAVORITE VERSE ABOUT FASTING:

Is not this the fast that I have chosen? to loose the bands
of wickedness, to undo the heavy burdens, and to let the
oppressed go free, and that ye break every yoke?
—*Isaiah 58:6*

Question: How did God lead your church into fasting?

Ayars: The first time our church fasted on a corporate scale
(churchwide) was for an assistant pastor's wife who had just
delivered a baby. The report came back that the child had spinal
meningitis, so we called a churchwide fast. It was just a day of
fasting and prayer, including several designated prayer meetings,
as well as times when individuals fasted and prayed for healing.

Question: What were the results of that fast?

Ayars: Well, the boy now is about 18 years old and he is fine.

Question: Were there other specific fasts?

Ayars: After that we started fasting from time to time for special needs. We have a friend named George, my automobile mechanic. As a young man, George got cancer and the diagnosis was very serious. The doctors essentially told him that he had just a matter of days to live. We decided to have a churchwide fast for him and pray for his healing. God healed him, and just a few weeks ago he worked on my car. He's in church on a regular basis.

Question: When you call a churchwide fast, how do you prepare your people?

Ayars: First of all I stay perfectly calm and I trust God for whatever answer He gives us. I don't trust our ability to fast; I trust God. Second, I suggest to the church members a particular day for fasting where we set aside that day for prayer. I recommend we fast from sundown one day until sundown the next day. God recorded each day in Genesis as the evening and the morning of the first day. So we begin fasting in the evening, then we fast breakfast, lunch and then we resume eating after the sun goes down. This is the one-day fast. I suggest that the people fast according to their own individual capacity. Some people are diabetic; other people have different health requirements. I tell them that fasting is voluntarily giving up food, or a kind of food, or all food. In some cases our people drink juices, in other cases just water.

I don't tell them exactly what they have to give up, but I point out the various ways to perform a fast, and ask them to let God lead them how they should do it. Usually when we call a corporate fast, we'll have prayer meetings in church, maybe at 6:00 A.M. for commuters, then we'll come together in a corporate praying meeting in the evening.

Question: If a person were to fast for the first time, what directions would you give them?

Ayars: I suggest three things: Pray and fast in secret. I would suggest if they were going to fast, whether they receive instructions from me or someone else, don't blow your bugle . . . that could be an entrapment of pride. The second is to spend great amounts of time in the Scriptures—read, study, memorize and analyze Scripture. The third would be to meditate and pray that God would honor the purpose of the fast.

≩ TAKE-AWAYS ⋹

Fasting is a spiritual discipline for all, yet a time
for God to work through individuals or the whole
church to give greater answers to prayer than could
be realized without fasting.

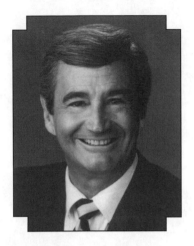

D. JAMES KENNEDY

Senior Minister, Coral Ridge Presbyterian Church
Chancellor, Knox Theological Seminary
President, Evangelism Explosion International
President & Speaker, Coral Ridge Ministries
Fort Lauderdale, Florida

D. James Kennedy is the senior minister of the 9,500-member Coral Ridge Presbyterian Church in Fort Lauderdale, Florida. He is president and founder of Evangelism Explosion International, which is the first ministry to be established in every nation on earth. He is chancellor of Knox Theological Seminary, and founder of the Center for Christian Statesmanship in Washington, D.C., which endeavors to bring the gospel of Christ to those who hold the reins of power in our government. He is founder of the Center for Reclaiming America, which seeks to equip men and women to work in their communities to transform our culture. He is the author of more than 40 books.

His messages are broadcast by television and radio to more than 35,000 cities and towns in America and several dozen foreign countries, making him the most listened to Presbyterian minister in the world.

Kennedy is a summa cum laude graduate and holds nine degrees, including the Ph.D.

26

LEARNING
THAT FASTING IS
FOR TODAY

Interview with
DR. D. JAMES KENNEDY

FAVORITE VERSE ABOUT FASTING:
In weariness and painfulness, in watchings often,
in hunger and thirst, in fastings often,
in cold and nakedness.
—*2 Corinthians 11:27*

Question: Do you practice fasting?

Kennedy: Early in my ministry I had assumed that fasting was an Old Testament practice and was not applicable to the New Testament. So I didn't fast. Later, however, I read the comment of Paul, "In weariness and painfulness, in watchings often, in hunger and thirst, in fastings often, in cold and nakedness" (2 Cor. 11:27). Paul's fasting caught my attention and caused me to investigate the matter from the New Testament perspective. I was led to believe that fasting was intended for Christians in the New Testament times as well. I then began the practice of fasting.

Question: Describe your practices of recent fasting.

Kennedy: My last fast was interrupted after four days when I walked into a few walls. I realized that I had started the fast too soon after a major surgery. I learned a lesson, and I want to pass that on to others, that there are times when you physically cannot fast.

Question: Describe a day when you are fasting.

Kennedy: Obviously, when you are fasting there are a number of hours of the day which are ordinarily taken up with all that is involved with eating, traveling to a restaurant or preparing food. When I fast, that time is available for spiritual exercises, such as reading the Scriptures and praying. The greatest thing about fasting is the extra time I can devote to my relationship with God.

Question: What do you eliminate when fasting?

Kennedy: My understanding of a fast, which I realize is not held by all Christians, is that when I have fasted I have taken nothing but water. It is my feeling that this is what is meant by a fast in the Bible, though some feel that taking fruit juices would be allowed. While I do not practice that, I do not disagree with their practice. I allow the Holy Spirit to guide each person regarding his or her practice of fasting.

Question: How would you suggest someone begin fasting?

Kennedy: I would suggest that those who have never fasted begin with fasting for a single day, and only after some experience would I recommend a longer fast. After a longer fast, it is important to begin eating very minimally as you get back into the normal routine of life.

Question: Have you challenged your congregation to fast?

Kennedy: As to fasting with others, we have on occasion invited the congregation to fast and pray, but never for more than one day. I believe that a corporate fast gives Christians an opportunity in a unique way to sever themselves from this world, and to fix their hearts and minds upon the world to come.

TAKE-AWAYS

Because many of your friends do not fast does not make fasting wrong, nor should you eliminate fasting from your schedule. You may read about fasting from these testimonies and then observe its practices in the New Testament, which is for today. Then like Kennedy, you may begin to fast later in your Christian experience. Then God can use its ministry in your life.

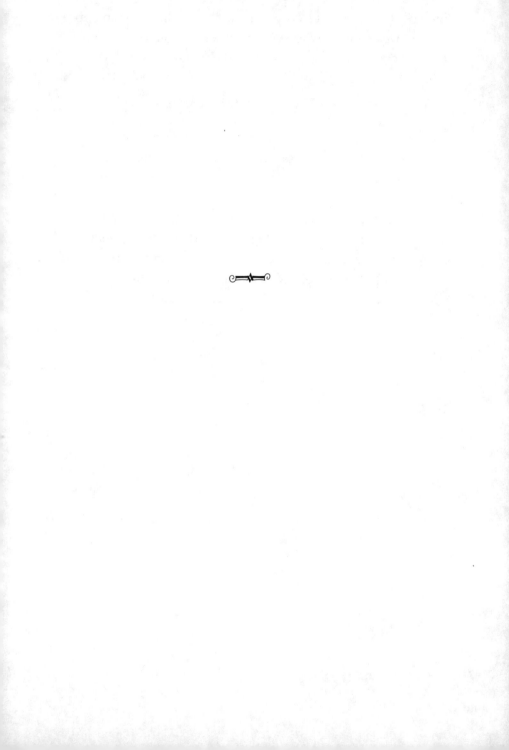

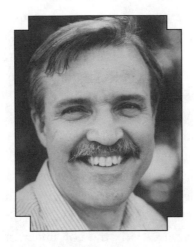

STEVE HAWTHORNE
Director, WayMakers
Austin, Texas

Steve Hawthorne is the director of WayMakers, a ministry focused on bringing about united citywide prayer that comes in close contact with the community. Hawthorne has coauthored, with Graham Kendrick, the well-known book, *Prayerwalking: Praying On-Site with Insight.* Steve worked with Promise Keepers to organize "PrayerWalk DC," which covered every part of Washington, D.C. with on-site prayer just before the "Stand in the Gap" gathering in October 1997.

Steve led a 40-day, 850-mile prayer expedition along California's founding highway—El Camino Real—from San Diego to San Francisco in the spring of 1995 to mobilize prayer and mission obedience. He speaks with living passion for the greater glory of Jesus. He says of his ministry, "I like to commit arson of the heart."

He leads the ministry WayMakers, dedicated to helping Christians extend life-giving prayer to every person on earth, and thus prepare the way for God's glory by prayer. Steve prepared a popular fasting and prayer resource called *Seek God for the City*, a 40-day guide focusing prayers of repentance and hope for the entire community during the 40 days leading up to Palm Sunday.

Before launching WayMakers in 1994, Hawthorne served with the Antioch Network as an advisor to churches endeavoring to start new churches among unreached peoples. Earlier, he served as vice president of Caleb Project and before that as executive editor of *World Christian* magazine. He is the cofounder of the research efforts among unreached peoples in Asia and the Middle East called the Joshua Project. Steve recently completed his master of arts degree in Cross-Cultural Studies at Fuller Theological Seminary's School of World Mission.

His book *Perspectives on the World Christian Movement*, coedited with Ralph Winter, has been widely used in many schools and training programs worldwide. He also edited the widely used handbook to short-term mission service called *Stepping Out: A Guide to Short-Term Missions*.

Steve helps churches cultivate maturity in intercession and research, and launching and supporting church-planting teams among unreached peoples. He has trained teams in on-site prayer in a dozen countries.

27

PRAYERWALKING

Interview with
STEVE HAWTHORNE

FAVORITE VERSE ABOUT FASTING:

He must increase, but I must decrease.

—*John 3:30*

Question: What is your favorite verse about fasting and why?

Hawthorne: "He must increase, but I must decrease" (John 3:30). This verse was spoken by John the Baptist, one of the finest fasters we have ever had in the faith family. Fasting is a way of diminishing the importance of clamoring desires and appetites. If I can send Mr. Hunger to the end of the line day after day, just about every other desire that God has formed in me can eventually find its best expression and true proportion. It's a way of gardening the heart, pruning and pulling weeds so that the internal beauties of "the hidden person of the heart" can emerge (1 Pet. 3:4, *NKJV*). As fasting is applied to seeking Christ and His greater glory, it seems to be a necessity of history's culmination that a people would emerge unseduced by their own desires. They would be unimpressed with their own stature and by the brilliance of their own love of His appearing, and move others to look for days of His visitation with eager expectation. And that's exactly what John did by his "fasted lifestyle." The results of his ministry was that "the people were in expectation" (Luke 3:15).

Question: What is the name of the book you wrote with Graham Kendrick?

Hawthorne: *Prayerwalking*. It has a subtitle, *Praying On-Site with Insight*. Prayerwalking is simply praying in the very places in which we expect God to bring forth His answers. We try to reserve the term "prayerwalking" to refer to intercessory prayer on behalf of others, rather than devotional praying.

Question: Can you tell me about the first time you ever fasted?

Hawthorne: The first time I ever fasted I think was for one meal, or one day, way back in my early years of following Christ.

Question: Did you fast for a purpose?

Hawthorne: I was fasting with some other people; it was to deprive ourselves a meal to engender a sense of compassion. It was poorly done, not effective.

Question: How do fasting and prayerwalking go together?

Hawthorne: Both fasting and prayerwalking are full-bodied ways to pray. When prayerwalking is done well, the entire body is fully engaged, along with the mind and spirit. Eyes and ears expand the range of perception of what God is doing and will do. The physical fact of our footsteps helps our own hearts to pray that God's kingdom will come in this ZIP Code as it is in heaven. When fasting is done well, prolonged physical hunger helps us recognize an even deeper yearning that will be unrequited until the Bridegroom comes in our midst again. That deeper hunger is our longing for Christ's manifest presence. This hunger is in the heart and soul of what we mean by revival.

I think it's best to finish fasting before moving into strenuous ministry efforts. Jesus fasted 40 days before beginning ministry. Is there a pattern or example in that? Perhaps we follow Him well by fasting first, and then moving into vigorous ministry. So when people are stepping out on a prayer journey, or prayer expedition (longer than prayerwalking around your neighborhood), they will be burning major calories all day long. It makes abundant sense to do your fasting beforehand. Actually, we usually find the fruit of prayerwalking follows fasting. You can couple the two together. First, accomplish your fast, break your fast, rejuvenate natural caloric patterns and metabolism, and then step out on the long prayerwalks or expeditions. But if you spend every day only prayerwalking a mile or two, I think the two could be done together.

Question: Three years ago you were involved in prayerwalking across California. Did you fast before that?

Hawthorne: We asked all 40 of our team members to pursue some kind of fasting before they began so that they would be refreshed in passion for Christ and would sense God leading before we stepped into the strenuous work of the prayer expedition. Two of our team actually fasted while they prayerwalked for much of the 40 days. I believe they were taking in water and juice, but no more. They were good for 5 miles a day at the most. The rest of the team were expected to prayerwalk 10 to 20 miles a day.

Question: What was The California Prayerwalk?

Hawthorne: It took place March 1 through April 9, 1995, the 40 days leading to Palm Sunday. We walked while praying the length of the founding highway of California known as "El Camino Real," which can be translated "the king's highway." The highway begins in San Diego and extends to San Francisco, in modern times often following portions of Highway 101. We sensed that the name "king's highway" had prophetic significance. But the historic significance is without question. Franciscan missionaries founded a chain of mission communities along the coastal regions, from San Diego to San Francisco, in order to reach the native Indian populations with the gospel. They aimed to establish a strategic chain of mission stations to bring forth a Christian civilization that reflected the kingdom of God, as they understood it. They wanted something radically different from the standard colonial life that had arisen in the rest of the Americas.

Question: What did you want to accomplish?

Hawthorne: We wanted to claim the best of this prophetic heritage by retracing the founding highway in prayer. California was founded for mission purposes, and has sometimes been the venue for great outpourings of God's Spirit. We are convinced that there is even greater destiny than good history. We aimed to catalyze sustained prayer for all of God's fullest intentions to come forth. It was a prolonged prayer of hope.

Question: How many people began and ended the prayer-walk?

Hawthorne: There were 21 people who were with it all the way. Nineteen others joined us for significant sections, so the team was 40 people. We walked it in 40 days.

Question: Were there other people who joined you each day?

Hawthorne: We called them "daywalkers," who joined us at specific points that were preestablished. Local people organized daywalkers who rendezvoused with us. They registered with us because we wanted everyone's name. We didn't want to have a tag-a-long band of people who had other concerns. We wanted everyone to be registered and walk with us as a unified body. We would walk together for three miles, sometimes as many as eight miles; then they had to get themselves back to where they left their cars. The core team would then walk on.

Question: What do you think was accomplished by this California Prayerwalk?

Hawthorne: Our short-term goal was to see an increase of united prayer within the communities of California. We designed the events and the evening rallies to model and to catalyze the prolonged on-site prayer in many communities throughout the state. We would never claim to be the source of all the prayer that God has aroused, but many people tell us that The California Prayerwalk legitimized and simplified prayerwalking for their church or city. Our long-range vision was the Palm Sunday hope of Christ being welcomed to entire cities, recognized for all He really is, bringing the glory of divine visitation. His "arrival" in divine visitation is all the revival that we will ever hope for. We believe we helped set the prayer agenda toward a fuller vision of Christ's greater glory.

Question: What else happened?

Hawthorne: The ancient route of El Camino Real led us through so much of what California is all about: From the slick banality of Disneyland and Hollywood to the powerful revival heritage of Azusa Street to some of the most fruitful farmland in the country to the tumultuous reality of the very active San Andreas Fault. Every one of these kinds of scenes evoked some powerful praying that we have seen God answer in part. We asked for huge spiritual harvest of the sort that we have seen break out in Central California. We asked for crime to diminish, which we have seen as well.

Question: How did you fast to prepare for this prayerwalk?

Hawthorne: I fasted for 10 days about a month before the prayerwalk. One of my personal intercessors had advised me to seek God by fasting without a lot of organization work for three weeks at a point about two months before the walk. With all the pressures of funding and organizing the effort, I made the mistake of cutting what could have been a 21-day fast to 10 days. Looking back, I can see God's mercy, but I would have been so much more filled with authority had I fasted as God had made possible for me to do.

Question: Was this a complete fast?

Hawthorne: I did a fast with fruit juices. A water-only fast would have diminished some needed physical stamina for the heavy exertion of the prayerwalk. Since then I have done a 21-day and a 40-day fast leading to Palm Sunday in preparation for other ministry efforts. I find that fruit and vegetable juice fasting need not severely diminish physical strength. Water-only fasting is wonderful for fasting for one or two days. I've learned that fasting is not to be understood as a hunger strike to force God's hand. Fasting is simply a way of affirming what is the finest value. By diverting every desire toward Christ, saying no to legitimate but lesser desires, we find all our desires recalibrated so that the dominant passion is Christ and Him glorified.

Question: Will fasting bring revival?

Hawthorne: Fasting is practiced revival as much as Sabbath rest is practiced trust. They are both prophetic. You are leaping into the end zone while you are still marching down the field. Fasting is not the opposite of the Sabbath rest. Jesus says, "You are going to feast on that day; why not fast now?" (Mark 2:19,20, Hawthorne paraphrase). Fasting keeps our desires attuned to Him. So great an affirmation is possible to those who fast by such a small negation. To say no to food enables you to experience the fullness of Jesus Christ. When you say no to food, you lay hold of God and grip Him with your whole being.

⇒ TAKE-AWAYS ⇐

Many disciplines are available to the Christian. This chapter focuses on the unique combination of prayerwalking and fasting, both ways to engage the body along with mind and spirit in praying. Several contributors use prayerwalking while fasting. Steve Hawthorne recommends prolonged fasts before entering extensive prayer journeys or prayer excursions. Find your own comfort level and do both as God leads you.

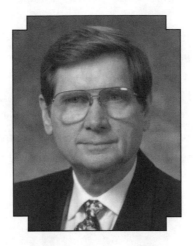

LARRY L. LEWIS

National Facilitator for Celebrate Jesus 2000
Retired President, Home Mission Board
Southern Baptist Convention
Greater Atlanta, Georgia

Larry L. Lewis is the retired president of the Home Mission Board, one of the largest organizations in the Southern Baptist Convention, which has a $100 million budget and more than 300 employees and 4,000 missionaries. Because of his extraordinary ability to administer this large corporate structure, and his great burden to bring revival to America, Larry resigned to work full-time with Mission America. Mission America is a group of more than 100 denominations and parachurch ministries committed to support and participate in the vision of Celebrate Jesus 2000. Their stated goal is "To pray for and share Christ with every person in America by year 2000 A.D."

Lewis graduated from Southern Baptist colleges and seminaries, earning his doctorate from Luther Rice Seminary, Jacksonville, Florida, in 1978. He has pastored several churches, including the 3,000 members of Tower Grove Baptist Church in urban St. Louis, Missouri, and was president of Hannibal-La Grange College in Missouri. In addition to these, he has held a number of state and national offices in the Southern Baptist Church, plus receiving numerous awards for outstanding service. Lewis has authored five books.

28

BUILDING
CHARACTER

Interview with
LARRY LEWIS

> **FAVORITE VERSE ABOUT FASTING:**
> This kind can come forth by nothing,
> but by prayer and fasting.
> —*Mark 9:29*

Question: How do you look at fasting?

Lewis: To me, fasting is just one of those disciplines that is important for spiritual power. At the same time, it is good for your health, good for your character and a blessing from God. In my case, it is a liquid fast. I have not eaten solid food now for 39 days. Through discipline I intend to keep the body under subjection. The essence of character is the ability to control your body and not let your body control you. The body wants to sleep, the body wants to lust, the body wants to eat . . . eat . . . and eat. Through fasting we can just say no to the body . . . you are going to obey me, I am not going to obey you.

Fasting is one way we can express discipline or control. At the same time, I do not believe fasting alone is the key to spiritual power or the only way to please the Lord. The Pharisees fasted regularly, faithfully, two days a week, and yet Jesus had great words of condemnation for them and their hypocrisy. Isaiah 58 tells us that even if we fast and pray, but are still living in sin, this does not please God. The greatest fast is when we keep our body in control, and fast from sin. We must fast from wickedness. We fast from being indifferent toward a world in need.

Question: What was the purpose of your 40-day fast?

Lewis: For several years I have had a tremendous burden for our nation as we come to the end of this millennium. This is the first time in history that our nation has come to the end of a millennium, and only one other time in the history of Christendom have we come to this point of time. It seemed to me that this was an appropriate time in our calendar to give the best we can to the greatest intensive evangelistic effort in history. Even more important than the calendar is the condition of our nation. It is in desperate need because of terrible decadence and sin. Not just me, but literally thousands upon thousands of people have begun fasting and praying for another great awakening in America.

I have been part of an effort called Celebrate Jesus 2000, which is seeking to get all evangelical Bible-believing Christians to focus on the simple goal of praying for and sharing Christ with every person in the nation. We want all people to be committed to their churches and to their church fields—not just to pray for every lost person in that church field. Then we want them to go to every door to meet each person personally—face-to-face—to hand them gospel literature and share the gospel with them. I feel like such an effort must be bathed in prayer. I am fasting to seek God's blessing in all this effort.

Question: Is it a coincidence that you chose to end your fast on the last day of the Prayer and Fasting Conference of 1997?

Lewis: No, it certainly is not. In fact, I started in 1974 fasting one day a week and did that for about 12 or 15 years. Then I let the discipline slide for a number of years, but when Bill Bright called the first meeting for fasting . . . the national meeting of religious leaders together in Orlando, Florida . . . I was one of the 600 there. He challenged us in that meeting to revive the discipline of fasting, so I began fasting again one day a week. I thought how wonderful it would be each year if I would precede that national gathering with 40 days of fasting and prayer and end on the final day of the event. This would be a good discipline for me. I am committed to doing that annually, at least through the year 2000.

Question: This is the thirty-ninth day; how do you feel?

Lewis: I feel just great. I feel strong, I am not really hungry. I feel some spiritual strength that I haven't had before. I went to my doctor on the thirtieth day for a complete physical and didn't tell him I was fasting. I just wanted to see what he had to say. He said I had never been healthier in the past 10 years. My weight was the best it had ever been, my cholesterol count was excellent, my blood count was excellent. He declared me in perfect health. I didn't bother to tell him that I had been fasting, but it just seemed significant to me that even the medical report was good. I can tell you for sure the spiritual report was good.

≡ TAKE-AWAYS ≣

> You can learn discipline and develop character
> through fasting. But fasting is more than saying no to
> food; it is saying no to all the lusts and sins of the body.
> Although fasting alone will never build godliness in your
> life, it is a discipline that allows your spirit the freedom
> to seek God and become like Him.

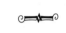

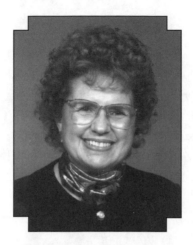

EVELYN CHRISTENSON

President, Evelyn Christenson Ministries
St. Paul, Minnesota

Although women and women's groups have always prayed, Evelyn Christenson is a pioneer in organizing women's groups for prayer in churches, denominations, cultures and continents. She had no idea how she would influence the prayer movement when she wrote *What Happens When Women Pray*. The book, published by Victor Books, has sold more than 3 million copies and has been translated into many languages.

She has been used of God to write *Lord, Change Me*, which has sold one million copies and has been translated worldwide. Other spin-offs are based on her pivotal book *What Happens When Children Pray*, also on *What Happens When God Answers Prayer* and *A Study Guide for Evangelism Praying* (43 languages), used internationally by A.D. 2000 North American Women's Prayer Track.

Evelyn is the wife of a successful pastor in the Baptist General Conference. She wrote her first book in response to a request by the national initiative "The Crusade of the Americas" in 1968-1969 to find out what really does happen when women pray. What she thought was a simple experimentation in prayer with the ladies of her husband's church Bible study has become a worldwide influence for God. Evelyn has held Prayer Seminar tours in 42 countries on all continents of the world.

29

FASTING
IN HER SPIRIT

Interview with
EVELYN CHRISTENSON

FAVORITE VERSE ABOUT FASTING:

I beseech you therefore, brethren, by the mercies of
God, that ye present your bodies a living sacrifice, holy,
acceptable unto God, which is your reasonable service.
—*Romans 12:1*

Question: What has happened in your life through fasting?

Christenson: Right now I can't fast. I was diagnosed last
spring with a very serious heart defect; something I picked up
overseas. They are monitoring how much water is going into my
body. I can't drink much water or liquids and I have to get
weighed every morning. So I have to eat enough to keep my
medicine down. I can't say anything current about my fasting,
but fasting has been a past activity.

Question: Did you fast as you wrote the book *What Happens*

When Women Pray? (The best-selling book by Victor Books, 1992, sold more than 2 million copies. It was the best-selling book in the United Kingdom for 10 years; these copies were not counted in sales in the United States.)

Christenson: I listen to God in my closet and I write down what He says to me. He brings Scripture quotations to my mind and I write them down. He reminds me of illustrations or circumstances in my life that can be included in my books. God brings all this to me in my prayer closet. I kept a notebook and prayed and fasted my way through writing the book *What Happens When Women Pray.* I wish I could say to you fasting was included as a section in the book, but it wasn't.

Question: Describe your fasting.

Christenson: It is more important for me to fast my time than anything else. While I used to fast from food, now God has called me to fast my time. I consistently fast my sleep and my nights. Obeying His command in Romans 12:1, I gave my body to God in 1965. But I took a sleeping tablet every night thinking I needed eight hours of sleep. Two years later, I realized I was taking it back every night, so I unceremoniously dumped the pills—and gave God my nights, too. Since 1967, I sleep very little. I never go to sleep until after 11:00 P.M. with my husband who is a night guy. I am awake by 3:30 or 4:30 in the morning and that has been consistent for all these years. It is during these times I get my praying done. In the past I may have fasted a meal in the day, or fasted all meals in that day; but now my time is the precious gift I present to God.

Question: Describe your time with God.

Christenson: Although I have given God all of my time, literally it is in the night when I pray, listen and write down what God tells me. It begins to fall into outline form, then chapter form and finally book form—all of my books and all of my materials are developed this way. I have given my time, my body, everything to God. This has been a complete sacrifice all these years, and yet has brought freedom and unspeakable joy through the years. Also, God honored it to produce my worldwide ministry.

Question: Why did you attend the conference sponsored by Bill Bright on fasting?

Christenson: I have been in the spirit of fasting throughout my ministry. It is my sacrificial spirit fasting, not just an outward bodily thing. I had been deeply agonizing in prayer 46 years for God to send revival to America when Bill Bright invited me to attend his first Fasting and Prayer Conference. I wrote him and said, "This time I am not allowed to fast because I have just had major surgery, but I will attend your fasting conference and I will fast with you in the spirit. I want everyone to know I support this endeavor and know it is the only answer to our country's moral and spiritual decline. I have practiced the spirit of fasting from food in the past, and now I want to be present and fast in the spirit."

≩ TAKE-AWAYS ≨

God does not measure the effectiveness of your fast by how long you go without food, or by how much food you give up. God looks at the integrity of your spirit. Those who can't physically fast can learn from Evelyn Christenson to sacrifice other things. Even though she can't physically fast, she attends the conferences on prayer and fasting to demonstrate her support, then she sacrifices her time, sleep and body to God.

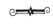

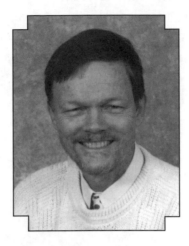

REX RUSSELL, M.D.

Radiologist and Christian Author
Fort Smith, Arkansas

Dr. Rex Russell is a board-certified invasive radiologist who practices in Fort Smith, Arkansas. A former three-year letterman in football at Oklahoma State, Dr. Russell now spends his time in the areas of vascular radiology, which uses angioplasty and other procedures to open up cardio-vascular vessels suffering from hardening or blockage.

Russell attended medical school at Baylor University in Houston, Texas, and completed his residency at the Mayo Clinic in Rochester, Minnesota. He has practiced at two of the nation's outstanding hospitals: St. Luke's Hospital in Houston and the Regional Medical Center in Fort Smith.

Being committed to biblical living for healthy living, Dr. Russell wrote *What the Bible Says About Healthy Living*, Regal Books, Ventura, California. He says that although a perfect, pain-free existence won't happen this side of heaven, there are tangible, proven ways we can improve our health and overall quality of life.

Dr. Russell believes following the answers to healthy living lie in obeying God's Word. Through years of searching for answers to his own struggle with diabetes, Dr. Russell finally discovered a successful plan for healthy living: don't eat anything God didn't intend for food; don't become addicted to anything; and ingest food before it is processed into unhealthy or harmful products. He answers questions about fasting authoritatively from a biblical point of view.

30

FASTING
FOR PHYSICAL
AND MENTAL
HEALTH

Interview with
REX RUSSELL, M.D.

FAVORITE VERSE ABOUT FASTING:

"When you fast, do not look somber as the hypocrites do, for they disfigure their faces to show men they are fasting. I tell you the truth, they have received their reward in full. But when you fast, put oil on your head and wash your face."
—*Matthew 6:16,17, NIV*

Question: What is a fast?

Russell: According to *Grolier's Encyclopedia*, fasting "is the practice of abstaining from food, either completely or partially, for a specified period." Fasting is an ancient practice found in most religions of the world. Traditionally, fasting has been a widely used form of ascetics, and a practice observed for the purpose of purifying the person or of atoning for sins. Most religions designate certain days or seasons as times of fasting for their adherents, such as Lent for Roman Catholics, Yom Kippur for the Jewish community and Ramadan for Islam. Also, certain events in the lives of individual persons have motivated people to fast, such as the day or night before a major personal commitment. The vigil of knighthood is a historical instance of this practice.

Question: How early in civilization did fasting begin?

Russell: Hippocrates, the father of medicine, used fasting to combat disease more than 2,400 years ago. The ancient Ayurvedic healers prescribed fasting on a weekly basis for a healthy digestive system.

Most think the Chinese, who originated four generations after Noah's family, have fasted since their beginnings. The earliest writings in the Chinese language are done on bones and pottery, dated 2000 B.C. These writings include stories of a seven-day Creation, the Fall of man, the Garden of Eden, Noah's flood and many other Genesis accounts. The Chinese also fasted, according to the earliest record of their civilization. Similar flood stories are found in over 200 ancient languages, including several Native American accounts. A word for "fasting" is also found in nearly all languages. The fact that the term for fasting is found in many languages would indicate that this practice occurred early. The origin of the fast may have come during the very Creation week itself. The seventh day of rest in the Creation week surely was a rest for the physical body, and may have been designed to rest the digestive system as well.

Question: How should a person prepare for a fast?

Russell: Several days before you start your fast, eat only things God created for food. Drinking pure water during this time of fasting is wise. During the first fast many people have a difficult time with withdrawal and hypoglycemic symptoms. The number of symptoms and severity may depend on the food addictions you have accumulated. Most symptoms will be mild such as a headache, weakness or irritability.

If you feel sick, eat. Then try to fast again in a few days. You do not get extra "macho" points by making yourself suffer. Next time you fast, extend the duration a little longer.

Try stretching the hours by eating lunch, then skipping supper. You will be sleeping during the toughest time of the fast. Then you *break fast* with praise for the food God has designed for you. Before long you will do 24 hours with water or juice only. You will feel great. Doing this once or even twice a week may be greatly beneficial to you. Later you can extend the fast to three days every month or two. Let God direct you for longer fasts. You will not be the first to complete a long fast.

Supplementing your fast with freshly squeezed juices and broths may be helpful. Drink pure distilled water. Even a partial fast with vegetables is beneficial. Avoid all chemicals possible during a fast. Seek advice for your specific problems.

Fasting is not a competitive sport. You do not have to set any records. Your body does not get healthier if you "out-fast" your friend or opponent. God does not give you a special crown for sacrificing more food than anyone else. There is no scorecard! Don't sulk if your spouse "out-fasts" you.

Most people who rely heavily on fasting for health purposes recommend an occasional weekend fast or even a weeklong fast. I can assure you that if you're healthy, this type of fasting won't be harmful to you. There have been numerous examples in human history of persons who have fasted (partial) up to 40 days without harm to their bodies. In fact, many have recovered from many maladies during times of fasting. Always end a fast by eating only real food (unclean meat was not designed for food, "You must distinguish between the unclean and the clean, between living creatures that may be eaten and those that may not be eaten" [Lev. 11:47, *NIV*]).

Question: What are some physical benefits of fasting?

Russell: Our bodies were designed to take a rest from food. One of the main benefits of a night's sleep includes rest for our digestive systems. In the English language the first meal of the day is named "break-fast."

Even a 12- to 14-hour fast can be beneficial. Some health counselors have taught that there are benefits to skipping the traditional breakfast and waiting until one gets hungry. Many like to do this, but they may get criticized by Mom, medicine and those who say we must eat three meals a day. Certainly weight loss would be an eventual physical benefit. Healing at the cellular level needs nutrients to metabolize food for energy plus the billions of other reactions that are carried on within a cell.

Note: the DNA has more information programmed within it than is necessary to program the course of all the galaxies in the universe. With all of the complexity of the cell, apparently it also benefits from time to clear waste products that accumulate.

Fasting is a process by which the body helps itself recover by allowing the body to eliminate poisons, waste and toxins.

Question: What are some of the other physical reactions that happen with fasting?

Russell: If one has food, chemical or other addictions, the first day may be very uncomfortable with headaches, weakness, irritability and even nausea. The symptoms may require the fast to be cut short. This short fast with symptoms does not mean that you are not genetically "cut out" for fasting. It just means you may need to supplement your fast with some freshly squeezed juices. Once you overcome the withdrawal symptoms a sense of well-being will accompany your fast. Hunger may be a part of your fast for the first 24 to 48 hours, but then your body gradually switches from metabolizing glycogen from the liver and muscles to metabolizing the fat stores in your body. Ketones are produced with fat or lipid metabolism. Ketones quell hunger. A very small amount of protein from muscle may be utilized. After the glycogen and lipid stores are gone, then protein is rapidly metabolized.

Question: Is muscle wasting a problem with fasting?

Russell: No, muscle wasting does not appear to be a problem with a normal fast. World-champion weight lifters use fasting during training and performance. Some Olympic wrestlers, professional basketball, baseball and football players embrace fasting as a way of enhancing their performance.

The source of energy during the first few days of fasting comes from the glycogen stores in the liver and muscles. Protein breakdown is not a problem.

The key to healthy fasting is knowing when to begin and when to stop. Jesus stopped fasting when He became hungry (40 days).

Irish protesters who fasted were carefully monitored. The protesters all survived more than 40 days. Once hunger began, if they continued to refuse food, starvation began and death followed within a few weeks. As far as health is concerned, the key to ending a fast is the body's signal of hunger. Hunger marks the beginning of starvation, which includes the rapid breakdown of protein in muscle and bone.

Question: What evidence shows us that fasting is healthy?

Russell: Your body was designed to fight sickness with a fast. Fever, fasting and rest are part of the design! Do you remember the last time you were sick? Did you want to eat? Did you want to party? No! You had a temperature, you could not keep any food down (forced fast), and you only wanted to crawl into your bed and be left alone (rest). Fever causes us to ache, sending us to rest. Fever also inhibits viral and bacterial growth by several mechanisms. Fever is good, but too much of a good thing can be harmful. A fever of 106 degrees can cause death or brain damage and should be treated quickly.

Question: Can you get relief from diseases by fasting?

Russell: Research by George Thampy, Ph.D, a biochemist at the University of Indiana, on 60 subjects who participated in a three-week-long water fast revealed significant observations:

1. Significant lowering of cholesterol;
2. Lowering of blood pressure;
3. Relief from arthritis;
4. Loss of body mass (as much as 40 pounds during the three-week-long fast).

European studies showed that fasters who were relieved of the above health problems and maintained a Genesis 1:29 (vegetarian) diet did not regain weight and were relieved of arthritis, etc., after a one year follow-up. Currently, Thampy is "chasing" a certain factor that is known to kill tumor cells. This factor is absent in tumor patients and may be elevated in fasting subjects. The immune system and the blood cells are enhanced by fasting; therefore, a wide range of protection from diseases can occur.

Question: Are there psychological benefits from fasting?

Russell: There are some mental benefits to fasting including a calming effect, the ability to focus on priorities and a generalized improvement in mental functioning. Don't expect mental miracles on your first fast. Addiction and withdrawal symptoms (irritability, anger, etc.) could override any first-time benefits of fasting. However, many soon learn to enjoy the discipline of fasting.

Even more striking examples of improvement of mental disease have been described. A Kansas couple, both of whom were physicians, had an autistic son. They discovered fasting when the boy was 12 years old. After a three-day fast, the son began to respond to them for the first time in his life. Through fasting, they discovered that the son had mental capabilities far above their expectations. The symptoms of many other mental illnesses such as hyperactivity, dyslexia, incorrigible delinquency, schizophrenia and depression have cleared temporarily during short fasts.

Question: What other mental benefits come from fasting?

Russell: The mind is a precious thing. Fasting can give the body time to clear the toxic products that can come from eating unclean, chemicalized or overly processed food. I also believe that eating things intended for food in their purist form is also great for the mind. Dr. Yuri Nikolayave, University of Moscow, a psychiatrist, treated schizophrenics with water fasts for 25 to 30 days. This was followed by a similar period of eating food in its purist form. Seventy percent of his patients remained free from symptoms for the duration of the six-year study. In patients with these advanced illnesses, profound biochemical changes do occur during the fast. Dr. Allan Cott, M.D., New York University, has used this fasting treatment on 28 schizophrenic patients. He reported a 60 percent recovery rate from this dreaded disease.

For many similar cases, read *Brain Allergies* by William Philpott, M.D., a neuropsychiatrist. He treated these food "allergies" by withdrawing the offending foods for three months. Pediatricians, cardiologists, internists and many other specialists use this form of unconventional treatment for many ailments with interesting results.

Question: Can spiritual problems like gluttony and addictions be helped by fasting?

Russell: Yes, fasting can be used to break addiction and slavery to food. "But Israel was soon overfed; yes, fat and bloated; then, in plenty, they forsook their God" (Deut. 32:15, *TLB*). It is possible to make food your god and become addicted to it, or a slave to a certain type of food. Oswald Chambers, in *My Utmost for His Highest*, states: "Make it a habit to have no habits." Even a good habit may keep us from serving our Creator. Food is good and necessary, but many people prioritize it higher than their relationship to God. "Don't let any chemical, food, or drink become your god."

Isaiah 58 reminds us that the fast frees us from bondage and breaks every yoke and is a wellspring of health. Fasting allows us to be obedient to the first commandment: "Thou shalt have no other gods before me" (Exod. 20:3).

Many things we do are good. Food, sex, work, etc. are all wonderful blessings if used under God's guidelines for their design. In my experience, these guidelines are best found in Scripture. The thoughts of God are the laws of science and nature (Florence Nightingale).

Other addictions that affect us negatively include sugar, fat and caffeine. According to Dr. Beasley's book *Food for Recovery*, these items make the body lose its ability to digest, absorb and utilize the few nutrients it is getting. If fasting breaks or prevents addiction, then nutrients designed for our cells could be digested, absorbed and utilized. When fasting is combined with eating the things created for food, this combination will be a "wellspring of health."

In general, fasting will prevent addiction to foods. Humans have imperfect enzyme systems (remember the curse placed limitations on the body after the Fall of man). Each person's enzyme system may be unique. This is why one person may be sensitive to milk and the next person can consume large amounts of milk without any problems. One person could spend a lifetime trying to evaluate how each particular food affects his or her body.

An addiction to foods such as sugar, salt, fat or caffeine will not be cleared by a 24-hour period of abstinence. Often food addictions require from three weeks to three months' abstinence from the offending food to clear the system. Regular intervals of fasting appear to protect us from a deficient or an imperfect enzyme.

Question: If fasting is good for us, why don't more people fast?

Russell: For first food fast, focus on fear factor! Phooey! Several years ago my brother told me how he had lost weight by eating only once each day. The rest of my family was fearful for his health. Later, when a three-day fast was suggested for my family, we all protested vigorously, thinking that we might die. I was afraid of fasting. Fear, I fear, is the primary reason! My fear was based on phooey! The Bible indicates that fasting is beneficial. Some other reasons people don't fast could be certain illnesses, food addictions, social schedules, peer pressure, and/or a lack of encouragement from the church, physicians, nurses, dietitians, etc. The Bible tells us not to call attention to ourselves when we fast (see Matt. 6:16,17). Many people are fasting and you will probably not know it.

We were encouraging our reluctant 13-year-old son at Astroworld, telling him how much fun the rides would be. His first ride was a spinning cup, set on a revolving undulating platform. With the centrifugal force of the spinning cup pulling our heads straight back, almost off our shoulders, he became very sick. While vomiting, his eyes turned to me and he weakly said, "Dad, I don't want to have any more fun." For the next few years fear gripped his face anytime I offered him "fun."

Strange questions sometimes get a strange answer. Fasting is sometimes glorious, sometimes healthy and sometimes sobering. However, if you have fasted for fun, you probably will not be lured into any activity that promises just fun in the future.

⇾ TAKE-AWAYS ⇽

There are many basic physical benefits to fasting. Medical research supports the positive physical results from fasting; however, any long fast or extreme fast should be done under the supervision of a health-care professional. But the normal fast of a short duration would be beneficial to most people. But, those who have certain medical problems or illnesses (diabetes, etc.) should consult medical advice before attempting a fast.

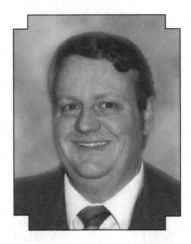

DOUGLAS PORTER

Chairman, Prayer Team
Parkdale Baptist Church
Belleville, Ontario, Canada

Douglas Porter has been used of God in a variety of ministries. As a young college graduate, he began Valley City Baptist Church in his hometown of Dundas, Ontario, Canada. The church grew rapidly and young Porter led citywide crusades for moral righteousness and against civic sins.

When Elmer Towns spoke at the church, he convinced Porter to move to Lynchburg, Virginia, to finish his education at Liberty Baptist Theological Seminary, where he completed the M.A. and doctor of ministry degrees.

Towns gave Porter a threefold goal to fast and pray: (1) to find a wife, (2) to lose weight and (3) to complete his formal education. God answered Doug Porter's threefold prayer. He married Sharan Livesay, a former college teacher and missionary to Brazil. He lost almost 100 pounds and he completed his seminary schedule.

Doug Porter has always been interested in church planting so he returned to Canada to plant Oakland Heights Baptist Church in Oakville, Ontario, in 1985.

Porter wrote *Investing in the Harvest*, a stewardship program for churches, published by Church Growth Institute, as well as *The Gift of Evangelism*. He also wrote the leadership manuals for the three "name" books written by Elmer Towns: *The Names of Jesus*, Baptist Publications; and *My Father's Names* and *The Names of the Holy Spirit*, Regal Books. In addition, Porter has been the research assistant to Towns for other projects. Towns said he chose Porter to help him write because, "I saw his sacrificial commitment to Jesus Christ. Many times when he lived in my basement as a seminary student, I'd see his light on late at night—studying. When he went to bed early, I'd see his light on early the next morning—studying."

31

LEADING A 40-HOUR FAST IN A CHURCH

Interview with

DOUGLAS PORTER

FAVORITE VERSE ABOUT FASTING:

Sanctify ye a fast, call a solemn assembly, gather the elders and all the inhabitants of the land into the house of the Lord your God, and cry unto the Lord.

—*Joel 1:14*

Question: What is a 40-hour church fast program?

Porter: It is a churchwide fast for spiritual renewal and national revival whereby members of a local church fast a weekend from Friday evening to Sunday. Whereas the Bible speaks about 40 days of fasting, it is very difficult to get busy laypeople who have jobs and complicated family lives to commit 40 days to fast. Because *40* in the Bible is the number of judgment and examination, we suggest a church fast for 40 hours to (a) examine ourselves spiritually, and (b) deny ourselves the pleasures of food. So we can sacrifice our normal lifestyle for the purpose of seeking God's blessing on our church with revival and God will renew our nation to its original purpose.

Question: What is your position in the church?

Porter: Steve Jones is the senior pastor of Parkdale Baptist Church in Belleville, Ontario, Canada, and I am the chairman of the Prayer Team, which is a group of people responsible for prayer in our church, and to be examples of prayer, and to lead our church in a successful program of prayer.

Question: How did you prepare the church for a 40-hour fast?

Porter: First, I shared the vision with the prayer team, knowing that all had to commit themselves to prayer and fasting. I applied the First Law of Leadership, which is the Law of Vision: "When a church buys into your vision, they buy into your leadership." When Parkdale Baptist Church bought into the vision of fasting for 40 hours, I knew that they would follow through with action. After the team saw the great potential, I presented the vision to the pastor. He bought into the vision, so we began implementing it into a program.

The pastor asked me to bring a message to the church on fasting. I preached from Isaiah 58:6-8, presenting the various fasts in the Scriptures. I used the book *Fasting for Spiritual Breakthrough* by Elmer Towns as my basis, pointing out the nine types of fasts. Technically, my sermon had 12 points and my title was:

WHY FASTING IS GROWING IN NORTH AMERICA

1. More believers are in bondage to demonic power, and God is using fasting to break that addiction.
2. Believers have complex problems because of the com-

plexity of life, and fasting is being used to solve problems.

3. Believers are in desperate need of revival and every tongue and tribe in the world needs evangelism, so the Church must fast to carry out the Great Commission.

4. Believers are crying out for the need of character and integrity in the Church and in our communities, and fasting is a step toward that answer.

5. The abundance of food in this world has isolated most believers from the reality of starvation and malnutrition in the world, and fasting will help us realize that humanitarian need and how to begin meeting that need.

6. The media has captured national and international influences of society, including believers, and they are living by principles alien to God's will for their lives, and that through fasting they can return to the will of God for daily living.

7. Even with the abundance of food, people are not necessarily healthier, but through fasting we can become aware of our need of healthier living and many in our congregation who need healing can receive it.

8. More believers are entangled with economic and social pressures that put them in bondage to materialistic goals, but through fasting they can be set free through the person of Christ.

9. Because of the growing influence of demonic powers in face of the declining influence of Christianity, believers need to fast and pray for the full potential of God's power in their lives.

10. There is a growing sense that each person in our society must take accountability for their actions and stop pointing the finger of blame at one another, and that fasting helps a person take responsibility for his spiritual and moral actions.

11. Many believers need to experience a deeper relation-

ship with Jesus Christ but fasting can bring the realization of His indwelling presence to their life.

12. There was a growing sense among believers that our nation has lost much of its heritage and basis for its influence, and a growing sense that we need to reclaim our Christian heritage on society and culture, but fasting is one way to bring national renewal and revival.

On the evening of that sermon, everyone was given a tract that I wrote, *How to Survive a Forty-Hour Fast*. After the sermon, I went over the tract, explaining to people how they could involve themselves in the 40-hour fast. The fast was set for April 3 after the evening meal through Sunday, April 5, until the Sunday communion service. People were told to break their fast by gathering around the Lord's Table (our church regularly holds communion on the first Sunday of each month). A bulletin insert was included as a support to the sermon. Also, Scripture verses were included to guide individuals in their study and prayer as they fasted for the 40 hours. There was an additional bulletin insert of an article "Proud Spirits and Humble Hearts" by Nancy DeMoss.

A commitment card was included in the bulletin, but because of the Canadian nature of the audience (Canadians are reluctant to sign a commitment), individuals were not asked to publicly indicate their commitment to fast for 40 hours.

The commitment card also included a response section for those who were fasting for the first time. It read, "This is my first fast, I would like a phone call during the fast from someone to encourage me in my fast." Only about 12 people requested help and/or encouragement.

Question: What response did you get to the fast?

Porter: About 75 to 100 of the 400 people in our church joined in the fast. We don't know the exact number, but that's how many responded in the Sunday evening service that was called "Concert of Prayer."

Question: How did each person fast?

Porter: Most people fasted from solid food, drinking only juices during the 40 hours. However, there were some who had physical problems, who fasted eating only vegetables. A few people fasted only one meal out of the 40 hours. I felt led of the Lord to fast during those 40 hours, even though I have diabetes. As a young man I often fasted, and fasting became a way of life. But after I was diagnosed with diabetes, I couldn't fast on a regular basis as I did earlier.

Question: Describe the "Concert of Prayer."

Porter: Approximately 150 were present for the evening service that was called a "Concert of Prayer." People divided into groups of 6 to 8 people, sitting at tables. We sang hymns of praise to God, and allowed for brief testimonies for people to share what God had done during the period of fasting. Approximately 30 to 40 people gave a testimony.

During the "Concert of Prayer," nine topics were given a short presentation. Scripture was read. When each topic of prayer was introduced, individuals in each small group were invited to lead out in prayer. After each topic was introduced, approximately two or three people led in prayer. On a couple of occasions, some prayed longer, took the entire time. The evening was ended as we read Paul's prayer in Ephesians 3:14-21.

Question: Where did you learn fasting?

Porter: I began fasting as a student at Liberty Baptist Theological Seminary in the early 1980s. I began to pray and fast for three personal goals that were given me, plus I remember Dr. Jerry Falwell, pastor of Thomas Road Baptist Church, challenging us to pray and fast for individual fund-raising goals for Liberty University. I remember one goal where Dr. Falwell challenged us to pray and fast for $5 million. There were a number of buildings on the campus that were unfinished, and we committed ourselves to a day of prayer and fasting. Dr. Falwell sent out an appeal in letters, plus announced it on television. In response to prayer, fasting and the appeals, God sent in over $7 million. The buildings were finished. This example left a permanent impression on me and my ministry.

Question: You mentioned three goals for which you prayed and fasted. What were they?

Porter: I was living in the basement of Dr. Elmer Towns's home, dean of Liberty Baptist Theological Seminary where I was attending. He gave me three goals to accomplish in Lynchburg. First, to complete my seminary education. I received the M.A. degree and later the doctor's degree. Second, to find a wife because I had tried to plant a church as a single man, and that did not work. I knew I needed a mate for ministry so I fasted and prayed for that period. God answered. I met Sharan Livesay and we were married July 25, 1981. The third goal was to lose weight. At the time I was overweight, and in a period of a year, I fasted regularly to know God, to get the answers to these prayers and to lose weight. I lost approximately 100 pounds of weight in that year.

꜒ TAKE-AWAYS ꜔

When individuals can't fast for 40 days, some can join a 40-hour churchwide fast for individual renewal, church revival and for the return of the nation to its Christian heritage. What Doug Porter learned about fasting as an individual, he translated into a fast for his local church.

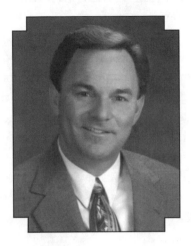

RONNIE FLOYD
Pastor, First Baptist Church
Springdale, Arkansas

Ronnie Floyd has gained a national reputation for motivating the Southern Baptist Convention to fast for revival. Even before being known nationally, Floyd was respected for building the large First Baptist Church of Springdale, Arkansas, from 3,790 members to more than 10,000 members and more than 500 baptisms a year—all this in a city of 35,000 people. The church has a $5 million budget, a Christian school of 800 students, and Floyd preaches weekly over the Daystar network, a television program broadcast over local stations and the FamilyNet National Broadcasting System.

Floyd has spoken at the National Pastors' Conference of the Southern Baptist Convention on several occasions, as well as many state conventions. When he preached to the pastors on fasting in 1995, they voted to have him preach the following year to the entire Southern Baptist Convention. God moved through one sermon to motivate thousands to fast and pray for revival. An audiotape of that sermon was mailed to all Southern Baptist Convention pastors, and a day of prayer and fasting was called conventionwide on October 25, 1996. A booklet and a book were also published by the name *The Power of Prayer and Fasting* by Broadman & Holman. Floyd has organized Awaken America rallies that have been conducted in major metropolitan areas across the South to call people to fasting, prayer and revival.

Floyd graduated from Howard Payne University, Brownville, Texas, and Southwestern Baptist Theological Seminary, Forth Worth, Texas, with the M.Div. and D.Min. degrees. He has published several books with Broadman & Holman, and has also filmed the video *Storming Hell's Gate*. He has held most of the offices in the Southern Baptist Convention at the state and national level, and is recognized as a leading revivalist in the Convention.

32

CALLING A CONVENTION TO FASTING

Interview with
RONNIE FLOYD

FAVORITE VERSE ABOUT FASTING:

Humble yourselves therefore under the mighty hand of
God, that he may exalt you in due time.

—*1 Peter 5:6*

Question: How did you get the burden to start fasting?

Floyd: When I was a college student, I became exposed to
fasting through some other freshman who pointed out the
Scripture reference on the topic. Then, out of a desire to know
God, I began to practice fasting and prayer even though I did not
even know a whole lot about it, nor had I heard anything
preached about it. I practiced fasting for numerous years. This is
what I call level one. Basically, this was no more than fasting for

one or two days at a time, but not on a regular basis.

Question: What is level two of fasting?

Floyd: I would say I began level two fasting about 1990 when my wife was diagnosed with cancer. I began to realize God was calling me to fast and pray for her healing. I began to practice fasting on a continual basis. Sometimes two or three days a week I fasted for her healing, but mainly one day a week, every week.

Question: What was the result?

Floyd: She was healed of cancer.

Question: Is there a third level of fasting?

Floyd: The third level began back in 1995. It came out of pure desperation of seeking the Lord. God gave me a deep desire to seek Him. I didn't know anything about Bill Bright's 40-day fast at that time, although he had just completed a 40-day fast. As a matter of fact, what God was doing in my heart and Bill Bright's heart he was doing in many other hearts, including Jerry Falwell's, that is, to go on a 40-day fast. I don't know if there is any history of God giving the whole Body of Christ a burden to fast, but I believe that is what is happening in America. This fasting movement seems to be from God.

I was reading the Scriptures early one morning when God made it very clear to me that when He told Moses to go on the mountain to pray and fast for 40 days, it was also my command. God made it crystal clear that He wanted me to do this for the country and the Church. I knew God wanted me to go on a 40-day fast for America and the Church. God told me that during the 40-day fast He would give me a message to preach to the world.

Question: Summarize the message God gave you.

Floyd: I believe the message is summarized in 1 Peter 5:6, "Humble yourselves therefore under the mighty hand of God, that he may exalt you in due time." God also spoke to me out of the book of Job, a message of repentance, brokenness over our sins, calling the nation to repentance. Today, very few preachers are calling our country to repent. I believe that is the message God gave to me to preach.

Question: After you fasted 40 days, how did God use you to call the Southern Baptist Convention to a fast?

Floyd: It happened in 1995. I went through the 40-day fast and then I preached at the Pastor's Conference of the Southern Baptist Convention. This conference is where most of the 50,000 pastors of the Southern Baptist Convention gathered. I preached a message from Joel 2 calling them to repent, fast and pray for God's blessing on America and our churches. I asked each pastor to fast and pray for spiritual power to influence their churches and through their churches to influence our nation. In that sermon, I described my fasting journey.

At the convention I was elected to preach the message on fasting the following year to the Southern Baptist Convention. I went through that year seeking the Lord about my sermon for the following year. I fasted often for my sermon; I had a year to prepare. I then went on another 40-day fast, really seeking solely one purpose and that was for God to send revival to America through the Southern Baptist Convention. I continually asked for God to put His power on that hour as I preached in New Orleans at the Superdome. I fasted 40 days for that one sermon, and God gave me the message I felt He wanted me to preach.

In that sermon, I called the entire convention to a day of fasting and prayer so that God might bring renewal to our country and revival to our churches. During the message that morning, God's presence fell on the audience. Revival is defined as when "God pours His spirit on His people." When I gave the invitation, it wasn't me or the human sermon. It was a supernatural intervention of God. The Holy Spirit came down. I remember Adrian Rogers came to me afterwards . . . hugged me . . . held me . . . tears flowing down his face . . . and he said this is the revival for which we have been praying. More than 5,000 people came forward, the aisles were filled and people couldn't get to the altar. People were kneeling everywhere; people were weeping everywhere.

Question: What were some of the long-term results?

Floyd: Johnny Hunt, pastor of First Baptist Church, Woodstock, Georgia, told me there is no greater movement in the Baptist ranks than what God is doing in response to fasting and prayer. Johnny told me that it was during that message that God called him to fast and pray for his church. In the last three years, no church in the Southern Baptist Convention has grown more than this church. It has more than doubled from 2,000 in attendance to more than 5,000. Johnny Hunt would tell you it is the result of spiritual forces, not programs or technique, but growth because of the power of God.

What has happened in Johnny Hunt's church has happened in many other churches. God is beginning a spiritual work in our convention and my prayer is that it would continue. If all our 50,000 pastors caught a vision of spiritual fasting and prayer, I believe the spiritual results would be spectacular.

Question: What other results came out of your 40-day fast?

Floyd: Through the experience of fasting 40 days and preaching the sermon calling for fasting, the organization machinery of the convention kicked in quickly. They got behind the momentum. Jimmy Draper, president of the Southern Baptist Convention's (SBC) Sunday School Board (the largest organization in the SBC), sent a letter to every church calling for a fast on October 25 of that year. He sent an audiotape of my sermon to every pastor, asking them to listen to the sermon. Immediately, I wrote a booklet, that was mailed out to 40,000 Southern Baptist churches, called *God's Gateway to Supernatural Power.* From that booklet came a full-length book called *The Power of Fasting and Prayer,* which was released last June at the Southern Baptist Convention while I was president of the Pastors' Conference. The books were written because of everything the Lord had done in my life.

Question: What do you think is the future of the fasting and prayer movement in the Southern Baptist Convention?

Floyd: I think some brothers have a problem with fasting. There has been some criticism, even though minimal, but, nevertheless, it's there. But we can't focus on criticism. I think some of us who have fasted and prayed and seen God do great works in our personal lives and churches need to boldly proclaim the results of fasting and not be ashamed of the power of God. I know everywhere I talk about fasting there is great reception to it. The reception comes heartily whether it is in a television audience or a seminary or in another local church.

I have preached on fasting at state conventions across the country. There is a tremendous receptivity to the spiritual potential of fasting. I think God is creating a spiritual desperation . . . a hunger among men of God to go to a higher spiritual level. We know we cannot change our culture unless God intervenes in a supernatural way. Some critics are saying that fasting and prayer are a couple of hoops we jump through in order to impress God. I don't think they understand fasting. Those of us who have practiced external or long-term fasting are well aware that if there is any flesh in our commitment to a 40-day fast, it departs quickly. It is hard to fast 40 days. You aren't going to make it if you try to fast as a legalistic maneuver, or as a work of the flesh. I don't believe fasting is jumping through a hoop. I believe it is God's discipline to fulfill 1 Peter 5:6, where we humble ourselves before God and constantly seek His face. There should be a continual seeking God's face through fasting and a continual humbling of ourselves to God.

TAKE-AWAYS

Fasting has great potential. One person can pray and fast for physical healing from cancer or he can pray and fast to bring revival to his denomination. Ronnie Floyd had to be revived first in the presence of God before he could be used of God to bring revival to the Southern Baptist Convention. We can learn from Ronnie Floyd to fast continually and fast for 40 days before great important meetings. The results of Floyd's 40-day fast are evidence that fasting works. But with every action there is a reaction; there is also criticism to the ministry of fasting.

FASTING
TO WRITE
A BOOK

Interview with

ELMER TOWNS

> **FAVORITE VERSE ABOUT FASTING:**
> Is not this the fast that I have chosen? Then shall thy
> light break forth as the morning.
> —*Isaiah 58:6,8*

Question: Why did you write the book on fasting?

Towns: As the senior consulting publisher for Gospel
Light/Regal Books, one of my tasks is to suggest new book titles
that are considered "on the cutting edge" or issues that are "hot
ones." In 1993—before Bill Bright started talking about a 40-day
fast—I recommended to Regal Books that they should publish a
book on fasting. As I was meeting with the editors, we discussed

who could write this book. We discussed several potential authors, but couldn't agree on the right person to write this book. I sheepishly put up my hand and said, "I can write it."

One of the editors asked the question, "What do you know about fasting?" It's a question I've been asked several times since writing the book. I've practiced fasting for 27 years, but I've never said anything about it publicly. However, I related to the editors that for many years I have taught a discipleship class on the topic of fasting to future dorm leaders at Liberty University. So they assigned me to write a book on fasting.

Question: How did you approach the assignment?

Towns: As I began thinking about the task, I was not sure I had enough material to fill a book. I had an assignment, but was not sure I could write a book—at least a book as long as Regal Books wanted. They wanted 160 pages; I was not sure I could fill 30 or 40 pages.

Question: Did you fast to get help in writing the book?

Towns: Not at the beginning. I began fasting at the admonition of my wife. Actually, I entered into a fast that I later would call the "St. Paul Fast," which is a fast for insight or decision making.

After I was assigned the topic, I told my wife I had to write a book on fasting, but I also told her that I only had one sermon on fasting, but didn't have enough material to write a whole book. She said to me, "Then you better fast about the book." Then she laughed, "You better fast about the fasting book."

I took her admonition and spent one day fasting for God's direction and insight about the book. During that one-day fast, I read encyclopedia articles, and did a word study on the word "fast" in the Scriptures. I broke the fast at sundown on Monday evening, and at dinner my wife asked me, "What did God teach you about fasting?"

My answer was simple: "I only have one sermon on fasting, and it only has eight points." Instantly, God spoke to me. My

answer to her was the outline for the book, and I instantly saw
the book had eight chapters. I decided to write a chapter on each
of the eight points in my sermon. I felt that insight came from
God because of fasting.

The sermon is from Isaiah 58:6,8, which gives eight practical
results that happen to people who fast. When I gave the sermon
to my students, I went through each of the eight results that God
would give them if they fasted.

> Is not this the fast that I have chosen?
> to loose the bands of wickedness, to undo the heavy
> burdens, and to let the oppressed go free, and that ye
> break every yoke? Then shall thy light break forth as
> the morning, and thine health shall spring forth speedily:
> and thy righteousness shall go before thee; the glory of
> the Lord shall be thy rereward.
> —*Isaiah 58:6,8*

My eight-part sermon was as follows:

1. "To loose the bands of wickedness" was "to break addiction and besetting sins."
2. "To undo the heavy burdens" was "to solve problems."
3. "To let the oppressed go free" was "for evangelism and revival."
4. To "break every yoke" was "to break discouragement and burnout."
5. "Thy light break forth" was "for insight and decision making."
6. "Thine health shall spring forth speedily" was "for health and healing."
7. "Thy righteousness shall go before thee" was "for influence and testimony."

8. "The glory of the Lord shall be thy rereward" was "for spiritual warfare and protection from the evil one."

Question: Is that the only time you fasted as you wrote the book?

Towns: Actually, no; my wife challenged me to fast on a couple of other occasions when I faced specific writing problems. Besides these two occasions, I determined that I would teach each of the eight lessons in my Sunday School class—one lesson each week, one lesson at a time. I determined to fast as I taught the lessons. I thought it was hypocritical to teach on fasting and not fast.

Question: Tell about one of those occasions when your wife challenged you to a special fast.

Towns: The problem was that before I began preparing my series, I didn't have titles for each fast. I was using a pragmatic or functional title for each of my lessons. I was going to use the lesson title for the corresponding chapter in the book. My wife told me that I needed better titles than what I shared with her. I told her I didn't have better ones. She said, "Why don't you fast about titles?" So I fasted the following Monday for God to give me titles. During my study time, I kept writing out different suggested titles. But none worked. By that, I mean nothing "clicked."

When I was breaking my fast, my wife and I went out to eat. She asked if I had arrived at chapter titles. All I had done was to study the functional or pragmatic titles, and had only rearranged the previous titles. I shared the titles with her, but she still thought the titles were too academic. She said they were suited for a college classroom, but wouldn't capture the public's attention. I told her that other than those, God had not given me new titles for each fast.

After about 30 minutes into the meal, my wife told me about a friend in the church who was raising money to go on a choir trip for ministry. Casually, my wife said the whole choir is on a "Daniel Fast" to raise money for the trip. When I heard the title,

"Daniel Fast," it electrified me. Immediately, I knew that was the answer to my fast. I took a paper napkin and pen, and began to write down a person's name with each title from the Bible lessons. I already had a Bible topic for each lesson. All I had to do was to assign it the title of the person in each lesson who fasted. Within a minute, I had arrived at the eight titles identifying them with the person in Scripture who was fasting. The titles of the eight are as follows:

1. The Disciple's Fast—to break addiction.
2. The Ezra Fast—to solve problems.
3. The Samuel Fast—for evangelism and revival.
4. The Elijah Fast—to break habits and emotional problems.
5. The Saint Paul Fast—for decision making.
6. The Daniel Fast—for help and healing.
7. The John the Baptist Fast—for testimony and influence.
8. The Esther Fast—for spiritual warfare.

Question: What was the other occasion where your wife challenged you to fast?

Towns: As I taught the series on fasting in my class, I skipped from Isaiah 58:6, not touching the material in verse 7. In 20 years of teaching my sermon on fasting, I had always skipped verse 7.

> Is it [the fast] not to deal thy bread to the hungry,
> and that thou bring the poor that are cast out to thy
> house? when thou seest the naked, that thou cover him;
> and that thou hide not thyself from thine own flesh?
> —*Isaiah 58:7*

After the Sunday School class was over where I skipped verse 7, my wife asked me why I had not included it. Plainly speaking, she asked, "Why did you skip verse 7?"

I told her I didn't see how verse 7 fits into my outline. The eight fasts that I had studied all had a practical application to the one who was fasting. But I couldn't see any application in verse 7.

My wife told me that verse 7 was in the Bible, and that I couldn't leave it out. Then she challenged me, "Why don't you fast to let God tell you what verse 7 means?"

I accepted her challenge. I fasted one day for the meaning of verse 7, asking God to be my teacher and to enlighten me. After the fast was over, she asked me what God had said. I had to tell her I didn't have an answer—yet. Approximately two weeks later, I was in my church prayer meeting, listening to a speaker from Mexico. He told about a missionary going into an Indian village in Chiapas, Mexico, to distribute Bibles to the unsaved, but had run out of Bibles. The missionary spent his weekly salary on Bibles to give to the unsaved. The prayer meeting speaker then said that the Mexican missionary had gone without physical food so that others may have spiritual food, that is, the Word of God.

When I heard that, instantly the Holy Spirit spoke to me and gave me my answer for which I had fasted. Verse 7 is not fasting for what you get from God, but you do without food to give necessities to others. I eventually called it "The Widow's Fast" because of the illustrations in the Bible where widows gave up all they had to give to others. We go without food so that we can spend our "food money" on other people. We give our food money so other people may eat.

Question: Did you fast for the book to be a best-seller?

Towns: No, I didn't think the book would be anywhere as popular as it has become (over 100,000 in print). I felt it would be a niche book that would be read by a small audience of spiritually minded people who were committed to prayer and fasting. I am shocked at the huge response in sales.

I thought Bill Bright's book would be a best-seller because its primary theme is revival, and that was a popular topic. The book's secondary theme is fasting. Bright's book is the challenge to fast; my book has instructions on fasting. It is much more practical, and designed to teach people how to fast.

⧰ TAKE-AWAYS ⧱

God will give you insight through fasting,
but the answer sometimes comes from Scripture,
sometimes from prayer and meditation and sometimes
from the insight of other people. We should ask God
for wisdom and help in decision making. We should ask
God to guide our thinking and creativity.

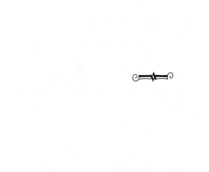

QUESTIONS AND ANSWERS ABOUT FASTING

1. Why should I enter a fast?
2. Must I always need a reason to fast?
3. How long should I fast the first time?
4. What kind of fast is best for the first time?
5. What should I withhold during my first fast?
6. Is it a fast if I don't completely abstain from food?
7. Is it a fast if I modify my diet to abstain from some food, while eating other food?
8. Should I have a fast if I have medical problems?
9. Is it possible to be neurotic and fast?
10. Can I fast and still go to work?
11. Can I fast if I have business or personal responsibilities?
12. When should I fast in secret?
13. What can I drink during a fast?
14. Is the 40-day fast possible today?
15. Can fasting be legalism?
16. Can we fast for more than one prayer request at a time?
17. What happens if you violate your fast?

18. Why are more people fasting today?
19. When have been specific times the Church has fasted?
20. What is gluttony?
21. What about second-guessing yourself once you begin fasting?
22. What guidelines should I follow to begin?

WHAT YOU WANT TO KNOW ABOUT FASTING BUT DON'T KNOW WHO TO ASK

The following questions have been compiled by Elmer Towns from his seminar conducted in a dozen cities across the United States. This six-hour seminar taught on Saturdays is based on his best-selling book *Fasting for Spiritual Breakthrough*, Regal Books, Ventura, California, 1996. During the seminar, people asked a number of questions. Here are the answers to those most-asked questions:

1. Why should I enter a fast?

You don't begin fasting for the sake of fasting; you fast for a deeper purpose. Usually, a person will fast for a prayer request that is extremely urgent or a prayer request too difficult to get an answer by prayer alone. God has given to us the avenue of praying daily to Him. He has invited us, "Ask, and it shall be given you; seek, and ye shall find; knock, and it shall be opened unto you" (Matt. 7:7). The word for "asking" in the original language is in the continuous tense; it means keep on asking. Sometimes you pray constantly, and the answer does not come. That is the time to fast.

2. Must I always need a reason to fast?

No, some Christians have made it a habit of their Christian discipline to fast one or more days a week. An evangelist at Thomas Road Baptist Church in Lynchburg, Virginia, fasted every Friday. Many people didn't understand why he was so effective in winning people to Christ. He got results that others couldn't get. He could turn almost any conversation into a soul-winning event. The evangelist never told what he did to get results, but he fasted every Friday for souls.

On some Fridays, he fasted for certain individuals, calling them by name before the heavenly Father. I am sure he fasted on Fridays for certain situations where he would speak or hold evangelistic meetings. He prayed, fasted and asked God to use those meetings that the lost might get saved.

There may be other occasions when you fast without a purpose. Many believers have fasted just to worship God. They do not have a crucial need, nor do they have a crisis in their lives. They have learned that God makes Himself more real to them when they fast.

First, you will discipline yourself to fast once a week to worship God. An individual at Thomas Road Baptist Church, Lynchburg, Virginia, set aside most Mondays to fast as a worship to God. He began at sundown on Sunday, eating before he went to church on the Lord's Day. During the church service, he began his fast, and after church service, if he ever went out for fellowship with individuals, all he took was a liquid to drink. This individual fasted most Mondays as an act of worship to God. It so happened that he was off work on Mondays, and could devote longer times for worshiping, longer times to reading Scriptures and longer times to meditating on the Lord.

Second, others will set aside a certain day to fast and meditate on God. One of the contributors to this book sometimes travels to the West Coast and gets caught far away from home with no meetings to be held. As an illustration: if he finishes a speaking engagement on Wednesday night, and then does not have another meeting until Friday, he sets aside Thursday to fast and fellowship with God. This fasting day is not for specific prayer requests, but just to fellowship with God, to worship God and to enjoy God. When fasting, he follows this sequence:

First, he spends time reading several psalms, specifically looking for those psalms that are prayers to God.

Next, he prays these psalms to God either in worship, thanksgiving or adoration.

Then he reads one or two Epistles. He does this with pen in hand, underlining the names of Christ, the key words of the book or some other item. Usually, Paul's letters have prayers, and he prays these prayers. When he is fasting, he also tries to read a large portion of the Bible about the life of Christ. Because Christ is our example, he wants to be like Christ.

Next, he prays the Lord's Prayer several times. Anyone who has heard him speak knows that he recommends everyone pray daily the Lord's Prayer, several times. (See *Praying the Lord's Prayer for Spiritual Breakthrough* by Elmer Towns, Regal Books, Ventura, California, 1997.)

Then he goes back through his last four months of prayer requests, asking God to give him those requests that have not been answered.

Finally, he surveys the list of answered prayers in the last four months. He keeps these recorded under the praise section. He uses these answers to prayer as a catalyst to worship God, thank God and adore Him for what He has done.

3. How long should I fast the first time?

I suggest you begin with the normal fast (i.e., going without solid food for one day). Don't start off with a 3-day fast, a 7-day fast and surely not a 40-day fast. If you start off with a longer fast, and something happens that you don't complete it, you will get discouraged and lose trust in your abilities. Then you have

accomplished the opposite of what the fast is for. You have weak-
ened your discipline rather than strengthened it. Start with what
you can do—a one-day normal fast.

4. What kind of fast is best for the first time?

I recommend that you begin with a Yom Kippur fast, which is
a 24-hour fast recognizing the way God puts limits on days. The
Yom Kippur fast begins at sundown the first day, and extends to
sundown the following day (i.e., 24 hours). Remember, in the
Creation God divided the days, "The evening and the morning
were the first day" (Gen. 1:5). So eat a small item before sundown
and fast the evening meal. The next day fast breakfast and lunch.
Then after the sun goes down eat dinner.

5. What should I withhold during my first fast?

There are several different ways to fast (See *Fasting for Spiritual
Breakthrough* by Elmer Towns, Regal Books, Ventura, California).
First is the absolute fast where you withhold solid food and water.
I recommend that you not start with an absolute fast. The absolute
fast is mentioned very seldom in the Bible, and it is usually iden-
tified with supernatural help from God (i.e., a miracle). It is impossible for the human body to normally function over a period of
time without water. The body dehydrates, and it loses brain cells.
To go without water is dangerous. I have known people who have
gone three days without, but I do not recommend that. I have read
about people who have gone seven days without water—probably
some physical damage was done to them.

I recommend that you begin with a normal fast, withholding
solid food but drinking liquids. If after several normal fasts God
leads you to a one-day absolute fast or even a three-day, make
sure it is the leadership of God. Make sure that you are not doing
it out of guilt or pride or to make a statement or any other reason of the flesh. Make sure it is the Spirit of God that is leading
you in this undertaking.

6. Is it a fast if I don't completely abstain from food?

Some non-Christians have done different combinations of fasts. One religion (not Christianity) will have a 40-day fast in which the people will not eat during the day; they only eat after sundown and before sunup.

Some Christians have been led to abstain from one meal a day, using that time to pray and worship God. This could be a valid fast.

A lady told me she didn't eat breakfast and lunch because she was fasting for her unsaved family. Her unsaved family had told her they didn't want her doing "religious things" like fasting to try to convert them. She did not tell them she was fasting for them during breakfast and lunch. She prepared the evening meal and ate it with them, with the intent of not offending, but lovingly attempting to win them to Christ. I believe this is a godly use of a partial fast.

7. Is it a fast if I modify my diet to abstain from some food, while eating other food?

John Wesley practiced what we call the "Wesley Fast." John Wesley fasted 10 days, eating only whole-grain bread and water. Wesley fasted primarily for his ministerial students. During this time, he was preparing sermons to preach to the lay ministers who were in charge of early Methodist parishes. Many of these men did not have an education, and John Wesley, George Whitefield, Charles Wesley and others preached one sermon after another to them. Then these lay pastors went home and preached those sermons to their churches. As Wesley spent his time praying and fasting, God reached England through these ministers. It was the beginning of the First Great Awakening that spread around the world.

The next partial fast is called the "Daniel Fast," where Daniel demonstrated that he could be healthier than others by eating only vegetables. Apparently Daniel didn't eat any meat, or other items from the king's tables (this might have involved alcoholic beverages, or even food that had been offered to demonic idols). In any case, Daniel entered into a partial fast eating only vegetables. On another occasion Daniel said, "I ate no pleasant bread, neither came flesh nor wine in my mouth, neither did I anoint myself at all, till three whole weeks were fulfilled" (Dan. 10:3). This apparently was a partial fast of enjoyable food, such as desserts.

8. Should I have a fast if I have medical problems?

Many medical problems would disqualify a person from fasting, such as someone who has diabetes, a pregnant woman, a nursing woman, etc. One medical doctor indicated about 30 pathologies that should disqualify a person from fasting.

God would not ask people to do something (fast) that would physically harm them. God never asks us to mutilate the body, mark the body or harm the body in any kind of aestheticism.

First, I recommend people who have a medical problem to treat their food as a prescription or medicine. They can eat during mealtimes, but commit themselves to prayer and join "in spirit" with others in the fast. When those who have medical problems eat, obviously they would stay away from delightful food, enjoyable food, (finger food) and only eat that which is basic and necessary for their health.

Second, I suggest that people who have medical problems make a vow to pray when they can't make a vow to abstain from food. God knows they physically can't fast, but if they pray as diligently as those who are fasting, God will join their faith to others for an answer. Through the years, I have talked to a number of diabetics who have the right attitude, who believed their prayers were just as effective because of the spirit of their fast, even though they ate enough to "accommodate" their medical problem.

Some believe they must "trust God" and stop eating as an act of faith and fast to God. Although they sincerely hold this view,

I am not sure I agree with them. I do not want to say that a person is wrong in leaving out food that is necessary for good health, but I want to tell them they must be absolutely sure their step of faith is prescribed by God. Many have taken that step of faith presumptuously, or they were self-deceived.

Because it is so easy to be self-deceived, I would counsel such a person to err on the side of safety. Eat a little to keep your physical health. I would counsel this person to remember the "law of silence" (i.e., when God has not spoken, don't make rules—for yourself or others). Because God is silent in the area of the sick person fasting, let us not make a rule to eat or not to eat; rather, let us recognize the physical mandate of the body; let us eat and pray.

9. Is it possible to be neurotic and fast?

Some people have a wrong attitude toward food. They believe anything that is enjoyable is sin, so anything they like to do must be wrong. They believe that because food is necessary and enjoyable, they are giving in to sin when they eat. Therefore, such people may think that fasting is spiritual, and just refraining from food itself will make them more godly. This attitude is wrong. It is not refraining from food that makes us spiritual; fasting gives us time for the heart to respond to God, and that makes us spiritual.

For those who are neurotic about food, I remind them of the great feast in the Old Testament. God's people were commanded to come to Jerusalem and celebrate the Feast of Passover, the Feast of Weeks and the other great feasts during the Jewish calendar year. When a Jewish believer brought a peace offering to God, the animal was roasted on the brazen altar and the Levite (priest) and the worshiper together sat down to eat an old-fashioned Georgia barbecue. They ate the food together in enjoyment and worship to God. (The sin and trespass offerings were burnt completely because of a person's sin, but the peace offering was a time of fellowship.) As a general rule, God made more provisions for feasts than for fastings.

As we come into the New Testament, we see Jesus coming to a marriage feast. It doesn't say He ate, but He probably did. He ate at the home of Matthew and Zacchaeus, and He ate the Feast of Passover with His disciples the night before He died. On several occasions Paul had a fellowship meal with the Christians, and in the Early Church they enjoyed a love feast before they served the elements at the Lord's Table. No, it is not wrong to eat. This is a gift that God has given to us, and those who say we should not eat misinterpret Scripture. Remember, Paul said, "Let no man therefore judge you in meat, or in drink, or in respect of an holyday" (Col. 2:16).

10. Can I fast and still go to work?

Yes, it is possible to fast and still work an eight-hour day. However, most people work around unsaved people. Perhaps it is not best to announce to your fellow workers that you are fasting that day. Remember the words of Jesus: "When ye fast, be not, as the hypocrites, of a sad countenance: for they disfigure their faces, that they may appear unto men to fast. Verily I say unto you, They have their reward. But thou, when thou fastest, anoint thine head, and wash thy face; That thou appear not unto men to fast, but unto thy Father which is in secret: and thy Father, which seeth in secret, shall reward thee openly" (Matt. 6:16-18).

These verses tell us a couple of things. Don't needlessly tell people you are fasting. Especially when you are fasting for a private matter. Rather, we should appear as we do any other day. Therefore, when you are fasting at work, ladies should make sure to put on makeup as they do on other days. Men should make sure they are shaven and their hair is combed so people will not know what they are doing. Why? Because you are fasting to the Father in heaven; He will see and answer.

11. Can I fast if I have business or personal responsibilities?

Yes, I have fasted and been called to lunch meetings and/or other occasions when people were eating. I did not feel any obligation to eat a meal just because I had gone to a business meeting in a restaurant where food is served. On other occasions I have eaten before I arrived at a business meeting, or my stomach was upset and I didn't feel like eating; therefore, I am not intimidated when I am fasting and called to such a meeting. When the server comes to me, I simply say, "I'll just take coffee."

I do not make a big deal of it and I do not explain to anyone what I am doing. I just take coffee. If someone asks why I am not eating, I say simply, "I just want coffee."

On one occasion I was embarrassed. I was called to the pastor's meeting of my church to discuss Sunday School issues. One of the older pastors sitting next to me heard me order only coffee. He said to me, "I've got plenty of money, I'll buy for you today." I just answered, "I just want coffee." The old pastor ordered a large garden salad with strips of sliced chicken breast. Then taking a knife and fork, he lifted a slice of chicken, placed it on a small dinner-roll plate and pushed it in front of me. At that time I had to explain to my friend, "I am fasting today." He was embarrassed and so was I.

I have gone to our church's banquets when I have been fasting. I had to be there because I am on the Sunday School staff. When the server brought a plate to me, I simply said, "I am not eating, pass me by." It was as simple as that.

At times while fasting I have had to have a meal, or in other situations I have had to entertain someone. When the other person was a Christian, I explained to him before going into the restaurant my commitment to fast that day. I asked him not to say anything. I tell the wait staff, "I'll just take coffee." I have found it is usually more difficult for my guest to eat than for me not to eat. When I see them put food in their mouths, it does not make me hungry, but I have found it makes them feel guilty to eat in front of me. So I try not to go to restaurants if possible when I am fasting.

12. When should I fast in secret?

You should fast in secret when you have a private request or for private worship. It is a time when you do not advertise your fast. Remember what Jesus said: "That thou appear not unto men to fast, but unto thy Father which is in secret: and thy Father, which seeth in secret, shall reward thee openly" (Matt. 6:18).

My pastor, Jerry Falwell, went through a 40-day fast through the summer of 1996. On the twentieth day, I noticed he was losing weight and asked him if he was on a special diet . . . again, or if he was fasting. Because I asked him, he told me he was on a 40-day fast and was halfway through. I thought that because this was a personal matter I had learned about by asking, I didn't tell anyone about it. The following Sunday, Jerry Falwell stood before the church and announced he was on a 40-day fast.

Many people in the Pastor's Bible Class I teach had comments to make about his fast. Some were not sure he should do it; some were concerned about his health because they thought 40 days was too long. Two people in particular were critical. They said that fasting was private, and they misinterpreted Matthew 6:18, thinking all fasting should be kept secret.

"That's wrong to announce it . . . ," one elderly lady told me.

"No," I told her, "you haven't studied both sides of the Scriptures on this issue." I told her that many fasts in the Bible were announced, especially when the fast was for a public purpose. I told her about the Ezra Fast, how he gathered all the people to fast, as did Samuel. What my pastor did was biblical; he was fasting for the financial rescue of Liberty University and the vast millions of dollars we owed. More than a year later, God magnificently answered the fast of Falwell. The school received a gift of millions, functionally eliminating capital-funding debt, although some debt remained on day-to-day institutional items. God had heard the fast of Falwell.

13. What can I drink during a fast?

The question of drink is debatable. When I was in Korea, I mentioned that I drink coffee during fasting. Many of the

Koreans were upset at my suggestion; they thought one should drink only water. On another occasion, I was speaking to a Southern Baptist associational meeting in a large Southern city. I mentioned that I drink coffee during my fasts, and one of the delegates was upset. From the floor he yelled an objection,

"Coffee is a stimulant and you shouldn't drink it during a fast."

My answer was very simple. "Yes, coffee is a stimulant and makes you more hungry, and if I had common sense I wouldn't drink coffee, because in a fast it will accentuate my hunger."

"But . . . ," my objector continued, "coffee has caffeine that will stimulate you physically." He went on to say we shouldn't do anything to stimulate the physical body, but rather afflict ourselves and feel weakness that comes by fasting.

I again agreed with my objector, but I pointed out the law of silence, which says, "When God has not spoken, don't make rules." The Bible describes that some drink during a fast, but it does not always tell us what they drink. On occasion it mentions they drank water. On other occasions it just says they drank. They could be drinking milk, fruit juice or other beverages (i.e., grape juice). They could be drinking just water. Then I said to my objector,

"I don't really like coffee. As a matter of fact, my secretary knows that I start on a large cup of coffee in the morning and it sits on my desk during the day. I sip it throughout the day. Sometimes I finish a cold cup of coffee after lunch." So I said to the objector,

"Coffee is like a yellow hound dog that just keeps me company."

Therefore, let me draw a principle about what you may drink during fasting. I think a person should not drink cola, milk shakes or all those things that we drink for enjoyment. Obviously, I think alcoholic beverages should not be taken any time, but under no circumstances should they be taken during a fast.

Some people drink only fruit or vegetable juices when fasting. Some think they should squeeze fresh fruits or vegetables because they do not contain salt or seasonings that are found in canned juice or in a commercial product such as V-8. A leading Southern Baptist advocate of fasting indicates that once a day he makes vegetable juice in a blender, then drinks that for sustenance. Drinking fruit or vegetable juice is not the same as eating and enjoying the chewing and munching factor. I like to drink V-8 juice on long fasts. Again, the law of silence applies here: When God has not spoken, don't make rules.

I knew an elderly man who drank a small can of Ensure, which is a balanced protein supplement drink to complement the diet. This elderly man did not eat normal meals, did not drink enjoyable liquids, but took one can of Ensure each day. Again, the law of silence applies here: When God has not spoken, don't make rules.

I have interviewed many people who have fasted for 40 days, and I asked them what they drink. People tell me they drink milk, Diet Pepsi, Slim Fast, grape juice and a number of other products. At one seminar, someone complained that Slim Fast didn't constitute a biblical 40-day fast. I replied, "Until you go without food for 40 days, and drink only one Slim Fast a day, don't complain."

14. Is the 40-day fast possible today?

When I began fasting in the early 1970s, I thought a 40-day fast was not possible. If you had asked me about fasting for 40 days, I would have said it was probably impossible. The only thing I knew about a 40-day fast was about those protesters and other political "rebels" who protested some action or movement and ended up in hospital beds. I would have said a 40-day fast was in the Bible, but probably not for today.

However, when Bill Bright phoned to ask me about his fast for 40 days, I cautioned him that at his advanced age he should not try it. Bill indicated he was going to be checked by a doctor daily, and he made a commitment that if the doctor told him to come off the fast for physical reasons, he would do it. I was sitting with

Bill Bright at the head table at a banquet in Wheaton, Illinois, on the thirty-ninth day of his 40-day fast. He had gone through Thanksgiving Day, cut the turkey for his family and sat with them for a lovely Thanksgiving meal. He said to me, "I wasn't tempted to eat once."

Yes, a 40-day fast is possible today. I, too, have fasted for 40 days. Thousands of people have joined Bill Bright in fasting 40 days for national revival and national return to the Judeo-Christian ethic.

15. Can fasting be legalism?

Anything in the Christian life can be done legalistically. Legalism is attempting to keep a rule for spiritual results. Therefore, we can repeat the Lord's Prayer legalistically, thinking that by the mere repetition of words we will become more godly. Or, we can give money to God legalistically. Legalism involves the outer obedience without the inner response of the heart. A person can legalistically stay sexually pure, yet in the heart be lustful and tempted to fornication.

Therefore, fasting can be legalistic. Some people have wanted to make a bargain with God. "If I don't eat food, will you save my husband?" This is only one example. People have asked for healing, money, deliverance and all other kinds of answers, simply because they fasted.

We can legalistically be baptized, attend church, tithe and do all the other things a Christian is supposed to do. However, just because we think our attitude is wrong, that does not give us the freedom to refuse baptism or to refuse to go to church. Rather, we must get our inward hearts right with God, then obey outwardly; that is God's requirement.

Because fasting can be legalistic doesn't mean we should never fast because of our fear of legalism. Rather, we should get right with God, approach fasting with the right heart attitude and withhold food for the right purpose.

16. Can we fast for more than one prayer request at a time?

Some think it is not a true fast if we are fasting for all the things on our prayer request list. They think it is not fasting if we have several prayer requests. In one sense, we usually fast for one compelling thing, but still pray for the other items on our prayer lists. A study of the original meaning of the word "fast" will give some insight. The word "fast" comes from the verb *tsom* (i.e., a word associated with emergency or distress). When a soldier is in the middle of a battle fighting for his life, he doesn't stop to have tea or breakfast. In his struggle he doesn't even think about food. In the same way, when we are struggling for spiritual survival, we don't think about food; we just want to pray and not even take time to eat a meal. That is the true nature of fasting.

Think of a man lost in a snowstorm, a family trapped in their van in a flood, or the time you heard someone you love had died. In the middle of the emergency, you don't think of visiting the hamburger stand to get something to eat. You surely don't want French fries or a milk shake. You want deliverance and you are yelling in your heart,

"Help!"

Therefore, the person who is fasting and praying usually does not attach all his or her prayer requests to the fast. In the true sense of fasting, we pray for one deep burden.

Some people do without food, putting themselves back into the mental state of an emergency. This is why the Bible associates "afflicting one's soul and body" (Lev. 16:29, author's translation) with fasting.

17. What happens if you violate your fast?

There is a difference between breaking your fast and violating your fast. You break your fast when you come to a natural conclusion. Many people fast for one day and do not eat until the sun comes up the following day. Therefore, they break their fast with a meal called "breakfast."

To violate one's fast is to eat during the time when you have made a vow to God. This can happen voluntarily or involuntarily.

I walked to my office manager's desk during the Halloween season. She had candy corn in a dish on her desk. I was fasting for a lengthy fast, and never even realized what I was doing. I reached into her candy dish, picked up two or three candy corns, and popped them into my mouth. After about the third candy corn, it dawned on me I was fasting and that I had just violated my fast.

I confessed to the secretary what I had just done. I retired to my office and confessed to God that I had not kept my vow to Him. Although not intentional, I had broken the spirit of my fast and was not willing to continue my fast. That evening I took a meal, and continued eating for the next two or three days. Then I entered into the fast I had originally begun before violating it. The second time I carried the fast through to conclusion. I did not feel guilty, because that was an involuntary action on my part.

On another occasion, I received a call from the president's office at the University, asking if I would take a visiting educator out to an evening meal. The educator needed to talk with me about accreditation matters, specifically about the School of Religion. I was on a fast at the time. Because the educator was not a Christian, I thought he would not appreciate my fast, nor would he understand my taking him out to a meal and not eating with him. Therefore, I intentionally violated my fast and ate the evening meal with him. Before the meal, I asked God's forgiveness and indicated to God why I was violating my fast. Again, I did not feel guilty, because I did the right thing.

Others have intentionally violated a fast. They just couldn't hold out, needing a hamburger or wanting to eat a meal with the family. Like all other vows that are made, the fast is a vow. Therefore, God gives a pattern how to treat vows that are not kept.

First, recognize it as a violation.

Second, ask God's forgiveness.

Third, recognize that we have hurt our self-esteem because we did not keep a promise we made to ourselves and to God.

Fourth, purpose to enter into another fast at another time so we can do what we have committed ourselves to originally do.

I tell people who have violated their fasts not to make a big deal of it. Confess it, put it behind you, learn a lesson from it and go on to the next event in your life.

18. Why are more people fasting today?

It seems a spirit in America is driving people to fast. This spirit of fasting has not been evident in America for the last 100 years. Richard Foster said no major book about fasting has been written in the last 100 years. I do not believe this book is a major book about fasting, nor is my previous book about fasting (*Fasting for Spiritual Breakthrough*). Why is there more being written about fasting, more talk about fasting and why are more people fasting these days?

First, because the Church senses a spiritual emergency it hasn't sensed in the last 100 years. America has been growing in military might so we have not been afraid of our enemies. America has been growing in financial prosperity. Our sense of ease and security no longer makes us afraid of a financial depression. America has been growing in materialism so people's lives have been made easy by modern means of travel; homes include every necessity and luxury for the good life; jobs include benefits, perks and security; national health and retirement benefits and the easy life are readily available. Having had no major threats in the past few years, fasting seems to have been unnecessary because few emergencies or distresses have consumed us. However, a spiritual crisis is arising. When we notice pragmatism, materialism, hedonism, demonism and false religions threatening Christianity in America, Christians are being driven to their knees to fast and pray.

Second, as the Church enjoys prosperity, we also are experiencing powerlessness, meaninglessness and erosion of commitment

and purpose. Even the people who attend church are less committed in their attendance than before. Christians sense that something
is missing: we do not know God experientially, we do not love
God, nor are we willing to sacrifice for Him. Therefore, to bring
America back to God, a few people are being raised up to fast and
pray for national revival.

Third, the light of New Testament Christianity is being extin-
guished in America. We cannot pray in our schools or read the
Bible. The courts are challenging the display of the Ten
Commandments in public, the manger scene in malls and other
displays of Christianity. Whenever light is turned out in a room,
suddenly it becomes dark. There is no middle ground; darkness
always follows the absence of light.

The gradual dimming of the light of Christianity is causing the
gradual growth of the influence of demonism and satanism in
America. Whereas America has been an outwardly Christian
nation, although not everyone is a believer, our outward commitment to Christianity has kept the influence of demonism and foreign religions out of our nation. Today, however, there is little to
hold back the tide of evil. So the Church realizes it needs more
than gospel preaching on radio and television. The Church is turn-
ing to fasting for spiritual warfare. Jesus said, "This kind can come
forth by nothing, but by prayer and fasting" (Mark 9:29).

Fourth, the collapse of character in America astounds us. It is
easier to tell a lie than to tell a truth. A boss tells a salesman,
"Tell them anything; we won't have it for a month." At one time
the public schools of America instilled character in our young
people. Character is still defined as habitually doing the right
thing in the right way. The problem is that we no longer encourage strong character traits; we don't know what is right. In that
situation, Christians need to learn discipline and character
through fasting.

Fifth, the abuse of excess may have run its course. During the
days of the Puritans, and even on the frontier, most Americans

didn't have much. It was easy to sacrifice and go without food, so we could give ourselves to prayer. The more abundance America has acquired, though, the more difficult it has been to sacrifice. Our abundance has become superabundance. Now, superabundance has become obscene abundance and sloppy abundance. Many Americans are getting tired of the phrase, "You can have it all." Many Christians want less; they want the presence of God in their lives; they want to simplify their lives; they want to fast and pray.

A sixth reason for the growth of fasting is the development of a worshiping church. Perhaps the best way to illustrate the growth of worship is to show the trend in what we have been singing. America was originally built on the great theological hymns of the Church that describe the depth of Christianity. Then in the 1800s, America was introduced to the revivalist music of Ira Sankey and Fanny Crosby. After World War II, the Church moved into gospel choruses where we sang our testimonies, "I'm So Happy and Here's the Reason Why," and young people went to Saturday night meetings to sing "Christ for Me."

Within the last 20 years, Jack Hayford has introduced us to "Worship His Majesty." We don't sing about God, but we sing to God and magnify Him in music. Our church services have become more than places to sing loudly, more than a place to hear the Word preached and more than a place to give our money to God; our church services have become a place where we can "worship His majesty." We sing to God, and now that we are focused on God, many want to fast in worship to God. Along with the growth of worship has come the growth of fasting.

A seventh reason fasting is growing today is that Jesus implied a return to fasting would occur right before He returned to earth. When Jesus was enjoying a feast at Matthew's house, the Pharisees began criticizing Him. They first went to the disciples of John the Baptist and got them to ask Jesus' disciples, "Why do the disciples of John and of the Pharisees fast, but thy disciples

fast not?" (Mark 2:18). Notice they didn't criticize Jesus for eating, only His disciples. Perhaps those who were criticizing Jesus
were bragging about their fast and wanted to know why Christ
wasn't doing what they were doing.

Jesus' answer was very simple. "When you have the bridegroom and it is a wedding, you go eat at the feast. But when the
bridegroom is taken away," and then Jesus implied, "and before
He comes back in the last days, then shall they fast in those days"
(Mark 2:19,20, author's translation).

Perhaps another reason fasting is growing today is that we are
nearing the return of Jesus Christ. Although I never tie fasting to
the return of Christ, I see a correlation.

19. When have been specific times the Church has fasted?

The Early Church fasted on Wednesday and Friday to prevent
any confusion with the Pharisees who fasted on Tuesday and
Thursday. Apiphanius, Bishop of Salomis in A.D. 315, said, "Who
does not know that the fast of the fourth and sixth day of the week
are observed by Christians throughout the world?" The answer was
obvious; everyone knew that Christians fasted on those days.

The Early Church also fasted on the days leading to Easter.
Over a period of time, those fast days have become meaningless
and legalistic. In modern days, some observe the fast of Lent, but
most who observe the fast of Lent do not do it out of a heart of
sincerity or anticipation for God to do something.

The leaders of the Early Church always fasted with a candidate
before ordination. The Scriptures indicate, "As the church was fasting and praying, the Holy Spirit indicated that they should send out
Paul and Barnabas" (Acts 13:2, author's translation). Then, the
"church fasted and prayed a second time and Paul and Barnabas
were sent out" (Acts 13:3, author's translation). From that occur-
rence, the Early Church tied fasting to the ordination of ministers
and commissioning missionaries. Although the Church has veered
away from that, perhaps it is a good practice to reestablish.

20. What is gluttony?

The dictionary's definition of a glutton is "one given habitually to greedy and voracious drinking and eating, a great capacity for accepting or enduring punishment."

Gluttony is more than the volume of food or repetitiveness with which we eat food. Gluttony can express itself in a "slavish" interest in the entire experience of food—smelling, tasting, eating, enjoying, etc. The gluttonous person is one who lives on the level of his or her appetite and is driven by physical appetite.

Fasting focuses our minds on the good things God has given us, but God has also given us food for health, strength and the enjoyable experiences of life. Those who don't eat properly get the opposite, which is illness, nausea and even mental problems.

When you fast, focus your mind on the good things God has given you. Remember, "Do not work for food that spoils," said Jesus, "but for food that endures to eternal life, which the Son of Man will give you" (John 6:27, NIV). While you are fasting, perhaps the Daniel Fast will lead you to understand how enjoyable a simple vegetable can be.

Fasting is not about withholding food, but about seeking God and His will, because the true meaning of spiritual hunger drives us to know God. Our hunger should point us to God, who satisfies. We seek God who makes our spiritual hunger go away.

21. What about second-guessing yourself once you begin fasting?

I have come across several occasions when people "rethink" their terms of their vow-fast after they begin. The most common problem is those who add additional "vows" after they have begun their fast. As an illustration, I have known some who have begun fasting, then they have added an additional abstention such as fasting from golf, fasting from television, fasting from sex with their marriage partner, fasting from attending sporting events, fasting from reading newspapers and so on.

Why have some people added extra vows to their fast?

First, they sometimes hear of how others have fasted from some additional items they didn't include.

Second, some feel guilty enjoying themselves while fasting.

Third, some didn't realize what they were getting into when they began fasting. When they got into spiritual warfare, they got scared, then upped the ante, adding a lot more items of sacrifice to their fast.

Fourth, some were not clear or concise when they began to fast; then as they took the fasting journey, some began eating things that made them feel guilty (i.e., cream soups and mashed fruits instead of fruit juice, etc). Others who didn't have clear fasting objectives and clear fasting vows began adding other requirements, such as one who told me he stopped drinking fruit juice because it was too enjoyable.

A fifth was a person who begins fasting for a request, but when there was no movement toward an answer, this person decided he was not doing enough, so he quit watching TV, no radio or CD music and no enjoyable walks in the woods.

As we look at these examples of those who have "rethought" their fasts, it seems some of their motivations have been "works" (i.e., doing something, or doing more to please God). Fasting should be motivated by grace; we can never offer God any bargaining chip to get Him to answer a prayer. God answers when we hunger and thirst after Him more than hungering after things in this world.

Others have "rethought" their vows perhaps because of a psychological weakness. It could be a weak ego, a negative self-perception or even some emotional problems. When some don't have the emotional strength to make a decision/vow, and to stick to that decision, they could very well change their minds about what they have yielded to God.

Finally, others have changed their minds about fasting because they didn't understand the nature of fasting when they began, or they weren't clear in their commitment when they began.

22. What guidelines should I follow to begin?

When you get ready to fast, use the following general check-list to help you think through the various things you should consider when fasting. Go through the questions and answer each one just as an airplane pilot goes carefully through a checklist for a successful flight. The following checklist will help you plan better for your fast.

≡ FASTING PLAN ≋

Purpose: _____

Fast: What you will withhold _____
_____

Begin Date: _____ Time: _____
End Date: _____ Time: _____

Vow: *I believe God is the only answer to my request and that prayer without fasting is not enough to get an answer to my need. Therefore, by faith I am fasting because I need God to work in this matter.*

Bible Basis: My Bible promise _____
_____

Resources: What I need during this fast_____
_____

God being my strength and grace being my basis, I commit myself to the above fast.

_____   _____
Signed   Date

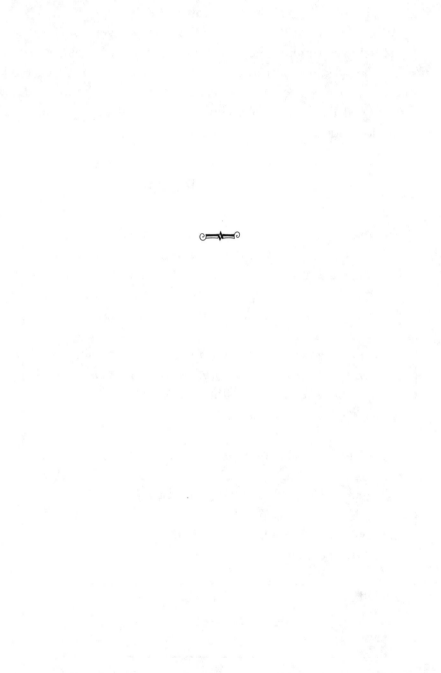

⇛ INDEX ⇚